Life After Epidemics

Life After Epidemics

Ebola Survivors and the Social Dimensions of Recovery

Kevin J. A. Thomas

Johns Hopkins University Press   Baltimore

Johns Hopkins University Press
2715 North Charles Street
Baltimore, Maryland 21218
www.press.jhu.edu

Library of Congress Cataloging-in-Publication Data

Names: Thomas, Kevin J. A. author
Title: Life after epidemics : Ebola survivors and the social dimensions
    of recovery / Kevin J. A. Thomas.
Description: Baltimore : Johns Hopkins University Press, 2026. |
    Includes bibliographical references and index. | Identifiers:
    LCCN 2025043724 (print) | LCCN 2025043725 (ebook) | ISBN
    9781421454146 paperback | ISBN 9781421454153 ebook
Subjects: LCSH: Ebola virus disease—Patients—Liberia | Ebola virus
    disease—Patients—Sierra Leone | Epidemics—Social aspects—
    Liberia | Epidemics—Social aspects—Sierra Leone
Classification: LCC RA644.E26 T46 2026 (print) | LCC RA644.E26
    (ebook) | DDC 616.9180966—dc23/eng/20250917
LC record available at https://lccn.loc.gov/2025043724
LC ebook record available at https://lccn.loc.gov/2025043725

A catalog record for this book is available from the British Library.

*Special discounts are available for bulk purchases of this book. For
more information, please contact Special Sales at specialsales@jh.edu.*

EU GPSR Authorized Representative
LOGOS EUROPE, 9 rue Nicolas Poussin, 17000, La Rochelle, France
E-mail: Contact@logoseurope.eu

This book is dedicated to the memory of Mr. Jeremiah W. Thomas

Contents

Life After Epidemics

1 Beginning Life at the End of Epidemics

Fear gripped residents of Monrovia in early 2014 when news reached the city that the Ebola virus had spread across the border from Guinea into Liberia. About four months earlier, an Ebola outbreak had started in the village of Meliandou, Guinea, near the intersection of the borders of Guinea, Liberia, and Sierra Leone. On reaching Liberia, one of the first towns the virus hit was Vonjamia, near its border with Guinea. As during previous Ebola epidemics, a major humanitarian organization based in Monrovia dispatched a team to Vonjamia to investigate whether these reports of Ebola were true. After the team arrived, including a young man named Blamo,[1] they quickly realized how bad things had become. In one community they visited, all the residents had died. Or so they thought—until they found a baby, alive, when they entered a house where an adult female corpse lay on the floor. As they drew closer, they found the baby nursing on the woman's breast, suggesting that the dead woman was its mother.

No one knew how long the baby had been there, but everyone realized it needed urgent attention. Blamo's boss asked him to pick the child up from the floor so the team could remove the deceased woman from the house. Placing the baby on his shoulder, Blamo carried it to their vehicle. As the team was preparing to leave for the hospital, Blamo noticed that the baby had vomited on his shoulder. Thinking nothing of it, he cleaned himself up and got ready to enter the vehicle. He was shocked when his boss stopped him to say he could not ride with the rest of the team. Although no lab test had been done to determine what caused the spate of deaths in Vonjamia, Blamo's boss was suspicious: Perhaps the baby was already infected with Ebola, and its vomit contained traces of the virus. In an abundance of caution, his boss gave him money to secure a private vehicle. Blamo traveled back to Monrovia on his own.

A week after his return, Blamo began showing symptoms of an infection. He was soon taken to an Ebola Treatment Unit (ETU), where a test confirmed that he was infected with Ebola. While at the ETU, his health rapidly deteriorated. He became temporarily blind and lapsed into a coma. Blamo was in this condition long enough for health workers to suspect that he had died. On the day a doctor stopped by his bed to pronounce him deceased, Blamo started to show signs of life. From that point on, his health improved. Eventually, Blamo was found to be free of Ebola. Before being discharged, he was told to expect to be stigmatized when he returned to his community. That turned out to be true, but it was only the start of Blamo's ordeal. Now, almost a decade after being discharged, Blamo still deals with health complications that make his everyday experiences more challenging than they were before he was infected.

With few exceptions, the experiences of many Ebola survivors during the 2014 epidemic in West Africa were similar to those of Blamo. They contracted the virus while helping others who did not know they were already infected. Today, their lives provide us with an opportunity to examine what happens to societies as they recover from epidemics. Apart from the fact that they survived their tragic encounter with a deadly and frightening disease, Ebola survivors represent many of the contradictions observed in the aftermath of epidemics. On the one hand, they experienced the triumph of beating a killer disease that threatened their existence. On the other hand, they face the challenge of continuing on with their lives in worse shape than they were before. As a result, they now risk falling through the cracks as they transition back into their communities, despite the fact that they took risks to keep many others alive in these same communities.

Such risks were not only observed in Liberia but also in neighboring countries, such as Sierra Leone. There, a young man named Tamba was enrolled as a medical student during the height of the Ebola epidemic in the capital city, Freetown. At that time, the surge in infections had resulted in the deaths of so many health workers that those who were alive hesitated to even show up for work. Nevertheless, Tamba felt that he knew enough as a medical student to step in to help, so he volunteered, along with two of his colleagues, to help treat Ebola patients at the Connaught Hospital in Freetown.

One of his colleagues soon started having diarrhea and showing other symptoms of the Ebola infection. Lab tests subsequently confirmed what they all feared—that he was infected with the virus. A few days later, Tamba and his second colleague started showing similar symptoms. Not surprisingly, both were found to be infected with the virus and were transferred to a special ETU constructed to treat infected health care workers. Tamba lay there unconscious for about six days. On the eighth day, doctors started to notice improvements in his symptoms. The good news? Tamba and his second colleague soon recovered from their illness. The bad news? His first colleague did not survive and became one of the many thousands who died from Ebola. When Tamba left the hospital, he expected to return home to a positive reception from his family, but that did not happen. On the contrary, it was the start of a long road to recovery that required dealing with a new set of problems he was not prepared to confront.

The West African Ebola epidemic, which took place from 2014 to 2016, transformed our understanding of the dynamics of disease outbreaks. For the first time since it was discovered in 1976, the disease spread beyond the boundaries of rural areas to urban centers in Africa and to two other continents. At least 10 countries reported cases of the disease—the largest number of countries with infected persons ever observed during a single Ebola outbreak. The most affected of these were Guinea, Liberia, and Sierra Leone, which combined to account for about 99% of all infections during the epidemic. Together, those countries documented a total of 28,606 people infected with the virus, the largest number of infections observed in a single Ebola epidemic. Collectively, the 3 countries also had 11,310 people who died from the disease. However, 17,306 of those infected survived. The largest numbers of these survivors were found in Liberia and Sierra Leone, which had 5,868 and 10,168 people, respectively, recover from Ebola infections.[2]

At no other time in history have such large numbers of people recovered from Ebola virus infections. Since the end of the epidemic, however, Ebola survivors have been forced to confront the reality that their lives have been significantly transformed by their experiences with the disease. These transformations are occurring in communities that were themselves affected by the epidemic and are now finding new ways to adapt to the presence of these survivors. Governments in the three West African countries most affected by the epidemic have also had to come to terms with these changes. In concert with international humanitarian agencies, they have been faced with the task of responding to social changes that have never been observed in their countries before.

For the most part, two types of responses are usually employed to address the issues faced by societies recovering from epidemics. The first is the *medical* response. Medical responses are an extension of the traditional reliance on medical interventions for saving the lives of the victims of humanitarian emergencies.[3] As such, they seek to address failures in the systems and structures that made it difficult to control the disease outbreaks that subsequently led to epidemics. Medical responses specifically prioritize interventions that directly or indirectly advance the use of clinical medicine to address the consequences of epidemics. Such responses include the use of foreign medical personnel to care for infected patients, the strengthening of health systems, the construction of new hospitals, and the development of new vaccines. Together, these responses address the immediate threat to human lives posed by viruses and promise to ensure that future outbreaks are contained before they become humanitarian disasters.

The second type of response is the *social* response. As the name implies, the main objective of social responses is to address the social dimensions of epidemics and their consequences. These responses include the development of policies to support those whose loved ones died from disease, to promote the integration of survivors into their communities, and to provide them with sustainable sources of livelihood. Social responses further seek to help survivors manage the long-term consequences of illness so that they can live productive lives in their communities. Additionally, they seek to strengthen the social infrastructure of affected communities, to invest in existing systems of social support provisioning, and to improve the ability of social institutions to respond to future epidemics.

What we have observed in the years following the Ebola epidemic, however, is the lack of an equal level of attention given to both types of responses. Specifically, the post-epidemic period has been defined by the provision of somewhat more consistent investments in the medical dimensions of recovery and less consistent investments in the social dimensions.

Since the end of the epidemic, new disease surveillance systems have been developed to increase the capacity to identify and track new cases of the disease. Shortly after the end of the epidemic, the US National Institutes of Health provided a large planning grant to four American universities to help them to partner with institutions in Liberia and Sierra Leone to improve research on viral diseases as well as to develop new tests and treatments for Ebola.[4] Today, at least three new vaccines have been developed to tackle the disease, and many more are under development, providing us with game-changing tools that could be used to respond to future outbreaks.[5] Some progress, albeit minimal, has also been made in improving the availability of health care in parts of Guinea, Liberia, and Sierra Leone.

Conversely, investments in the social dimensions of recovery have been minimal. Ebola survivors still live with the hardships associated with their prior infections, lack access to the resources needed to rebuild their lives, and face challenges to social integration into their communities. Additionally, they have experienced limited investments in the social dimensions of their health. As a result, survivors continue to struggle with disabilities associated with the long-term health consequences of Ebola, lack of access to affordable health care, and the challenges of living with physical limitations that affect their ability to work. For these survivors, the consequences of the underinvestment in social responses have been daunting. As a result, they have had to adapt to the new realities that have followed their recovery in an environment characterized by a distinct lack of attention to the development of sound social policies.

Survivor Narratives and the Significance of Social Response

This book addresses the implications of this comparative lack of attention given to the social consequences of the Ebola epidemic. Focusing on the lives of Ebola survivors, it demonstrates the continued significance of the social consequences of the epidemic to make a general case for why investments in social responses are still needed. To make this point, the analysis focuses on Ebola survivors in Liberia and Sierra Leone, the two countries with the largest numbers of people who recovered from the disease during the 2014 epidemic. Specifically, it relies on the data collected from interviews conducted with 250 of these survivors from 2021 to 2022; 100 of these interviews were conducted in Liberia, and 150 were conducted in Sierra Leone.[6]

Restricting the focus to these two countries allows this book to leverage the unique circumstances found in each setting and the respective resources each country had available for conducting the study. The Liberia sample, for example, focused exclusively on residents in Monrovia, its capital city, the majority of whom lived in poor slum communities found in an area referred to as Sector 2, as well as other poor communities. Similarly, the Sierra Leone sample included residents in marginalized communities in Freetown. However, it also included a small rural sample of about 30 Ebola survivors who were interviewed in villages in the Moyamba district, which was significantly affected by the epidemic.[7]

While Liberia and Sierra Leone have similar social histories and, in some cases, common political-economic circumstances, they also differ in ways that are important for understanding their respective experiences. For example, as noted earlier, the number of Ebola survivors in the former was smaller than in the latter. Health expenditures as a percentage of gross domestic product (GDP) were also lower in Liberia than in Sierra Leone just after the end of the epidemic.[8] Corresponding similarities and differences can also be observed in the experiences of survivors in both countries. The similarities are extensive, as will be shown in the common experiences found in the accounts of survivors in both countries. However, the book also highlights important differences between the two, in terms of issues such as survivors' access to health care, the intervention of local leaders to help Ebola survivors transition into their communities, and the politicization of relief aid after the epidemic.

Narratives collected from the interviews are the main tools used to develop insights into the experiences of Ebola survivors. Some of these survivors were leaders of various Ebola survivor groups who provided critical information about their members and about their relationships with governmental and nongovernmental institutions. Information collected from the interviews was supplemented with data from secondary sources. These included archival sources containing news articles published during the epidemic and its immediate aftermath, government documents in Liberia and Sierra Leone, and documents from international organizations such as the World Health Organization (WHO).

Using information collected from these sources, the book makes three specific arguments to underscore the continuing significance of the social consequences of the epidemic. First, it argues that, with few exceptions, the social consequences of the epidemic faced by Ebola survivors are not merely short-term limitations that will disappear over time. Instead, they are long-term challenges that have contributed to major transformations in survivors' life circumstances. These transformations affect not only how families are now configured but also the extent to which they can support themselves. Many of these challenges have been discounted in the traditional approaches used to address the aftermath of epidemics. This, the book argues, is in part due to a greater emphasis on medical responses, especially those that advance the use of clinical medicine and tend to end shortly after the end of epidemics. By contrast, social responses, which require an extended level of commitment, have been deemphasized.

The book's second argument is that, within contexts of recovery, social structure plays a major role in accentuating the disadvantage of Ebola survivors who were already from marginalized groups. Pre-epidemic social class differences that created disparities in susceptibility to the Ebola virus infection have thus provided a critical mechanism for reproducing inequalities in the outcomes of Ebola survivors. Survivors from socially marginalized groups, the book argues, have been pushed further down into socioeconomic disadvantage and face more obstacles to their recovery compared to their counterparts who had not previously been marginalized, including Ebola survivors in the West. This process has been facilitated by the tendency of NGOs to focus on the provision of emergency relief assistance rather than on strategies that advance economic development. As a result, important opportunities have been missed for improving the welfare of marginalized groups that already lived in poverty before the epidemic. Rather than experiencing social recovery, Ebola survivors from these groups have seen an effective reversal of their fortunes, making them even more dependent on others than they were before.

Finally, the book argues that despite the daunting challenges survivors face on the road to recovery, they still play an integral role in shaping the social problems they continue to experience in their communities. In other words, their tragic experiences with illness have been incorporated into meaning-making processes that have helped them develop a new sense of purpose and, in some cases, resulted in a positive reinterpretation of their experiences with the disease. To be clear, this is not a deterministic argument that holds Ebola survivors responsible for their welfare. Rather, it is a recognition of the fact that, even in low-resource contexts, survivors can find ways of adapting to their circumstances and navigating the complex social challenges they face in ways that allow them to thrive in their communities.

Epidemics, Social Disruptions, and Their Consequences

For much of human history, epidemics have contributed to a vast array of social changes in the places where they occur. Following the end of the Plague of Athens, for example, which took place from 430 to 427 BC, Thucydides provided a picture of the problems faced by an Athenian society that was attempting to emerge from the crisis.[9] Weakened by the massive loss of lives, it was incapable of marshaling its war machinery to effectively counter the threat posed by its enemies. One unit specializing in heavy machinery, for example, lost about 25% of its soldiers to the epidemic. Beyond the defense establishment, the city also experienced other types of challenges. These included a breakdown of law and order and a disregard for social norms. Indeed, the social decline that followed the end of the epidemic was believed to be the driving force that led to a collapse of morality. There is no doubt that these social challenges were significant. However, we know comparatively less about the lives of survivors of the plague, perhaps because their experiences are subsumed in the record of the broader societal disruptions.

Following the end of most contemporary epidemics, there is a declining level of attention given to the lives of the affected that becomes even more apparent with the passage of time. Media coverage declines, commentaries on the implications of these outbreaks become less frequent, and aid workers pack their bags and return home. While things are assumed to have returned to normal, societies emerging from epidemics cannot simply return to the way things were before these crises. As observed after the Plague of Athens, communities in recovery face a long list of problems that can pose a significant threat to social stability.

After the West African Ebola epidemic, the most affected countries faced similar problems, which were linked to associated disruptions that touched every facet of their societies. The most important of these, of course, were the thousands of people who lost their lives to the disease. Among them were health care personnel, including physicians and other medical specialists. Estimates indicate that 8.2% of all doctors died from the disease in Sierra Leone, a country that had only 134 doctors at the time of the epidemic.[10] A similar percentage of doctors is estimated to have died from Ebola in neighboring Liberia.[11] Given the fact that both of these countries had fewer than one doctor per thousand of their people during the epidemic, any loss of the small numbers that were available should be considered substantial.[12]

Not surprisingly, the loss of health care personnel was accompanied by declines in other health outcomes. For example, maternal mortality levels increased by 38% in Guinea and 111% in Liberia, while the reduction of malaria care due to the focus on the epidemic resulted in more than 10,000 additional deaths.[13] In Guinea, Liberia, and Sierra Leone, estimates also suggest that essential childhood vaccinations were given less frequently. As a result, hundreds of thousands of children were exposed to measles and other infectious diseases.[14]

This secondary health crisis that followed the epidemic was the result of other factors as well. Declines in the availability of primary health care were observed as major health providers focused on interventions that helped to stop the spread of the virus. Small and private health care providers were shut down, either because they wanted to reduce the likelihood of transmission within their institutions or because of staff shortages. Under these circumstances, the maternal mortality increases observed in the affected countries were not surprising, given the corresponding declines in services such as emergency obstetric surgeries.[15] In Macenta, Guinea, near where the first documented case of the Ebola virus during the epidemic was found, attendance at the town's primary antenatal clinic declined by more than 40%, while the number of HIV tests conducted declined by almost 50%.[16] Overall, the negative impacts of the secondary health crisis contributed to an increase in non-Ebola deaths, which added to the problems faced by the affected countries at the end of the crisis.

Social relations were similarly disrupted as the historical basis of community life in the affected countries became increasingly challenged by fears of infection. Traditional values of burden sharing, risk mitigation, and communal responses to tragedy were abandoned as the fear of Ebola spread through communities in the region. Once-friendly community members feared to participate in simple social interactions, such as the shaking of hands, as well as other forms of physical interaction that were central to the work of those who cared for the sick or buried the dead.[17]

Subsequent years have seen the end of the worst of these disruptions. Yet the vestiges of the crisis continue to live on and constrain attempts to return to normal. While interruptions to health services have ended, more time is required to replace the expertise of health care workers lost in the epidemic. Similarly, although social relations have somewhat improved since the end of the epidemic, the fear of Ebola continues to determine the level of social interactions survivors have with residents of their communities.

Societies recovering from epidemics have wrestled with these kinds of issues in different ways. In these contexts, governments typically look to rebound from the effects of widespread mortality on their ability to restart their basic functions. Systems for providing support to orphans and widows need to be strengthened, preparing for the possibility that they may need assistance over the long term. Government officials also need to consider larger structural shifts. Temporal changes in the allocation of labor, which were needed to provide an urgent response to the crisis, need to be reversed. Educational institutions closed during quarantines need to be reopened at the same time that plans are made to replace teachers who lost their lives to disease. All this must be done without losing sight of the need to rebuild health care institutions. After all, the rebuilding of these institutions is essential for screening patients with symptoms that could signal the start of another epidemic.

Unfortunately, as the needs multiply, so also does fatigue. As such, when the Ebola epidemic ended, so did the work of humanitarian organizations that shifted their focus to other global crises. While these shifts define how most global institutions respond to epidemics, they are inconsistent with the ways in which societies operate. Societies are organized in ways that involve a continuous process of change, and this change occurs regardless of whether or not it is acknowledged. As such, the fact that less attention is given to the social consequences of epidemics does not stop these consequences from being observed in communities. Partly because these changes are observed over long periods of time, it is easy to ignore their significance for understanding the lifecycle of epidemics. However, they raise important questions about the viability of the new social order they tend to engender. Past attempts to understand these issues have generated a wealth of knowledge about what happens to societies in the aftermath of epidemics.

Lessons from Contemporary Epidemics

Contemporary epidemics, however, create a new set of circumstances for improving knowledge about the societal changes that follow their conclusion. For starters, contemporary epidemics occur in an era of unprecedented levels of globalization. Epidemics today can affect more countries simultaneously and put more lives at risk than they have at any other point in history. Studies on their aftermath can thus help us understand these consequences in an increasingly globalized world. Emerging and reemerging infectious diseases further increase the likelihood that epidemics will become more frequent in the future. Therefore, it is important to understand the challenges that follow modern epidemics to better prepare to respond to them when they occur. Few cases are as important for developing these insights as that provided by the 2014 Ebola epidemic.

Nothing underscores the importance of these insights as much as what the world experienced in the wake of the crisis. Approximately four years after it ended, the Ebola epidemic was followed by one of the largest disease outbreaks observed in recent years. Toward the end of 2019, what started as a local outbreak of the severe acute respiratory syndrome coronavirus 2 (SARS-Cov-2) soon became the global COVID-19 pandemic, which affected more countries and people than the Ebola crisis. Many differences exist between the two global crises, including disparities in the number of people they affected. However, there are enough similarities between them to suggest that we can learn important lessons from the Ebola epidemic as we prepare to deal with the long-term social consequences of COVID-19. For example, both outbreaks were disproportionately more likely to affect people from lower socioeconomic groups. Additionally, the emerging evidence from people recovering from COVID-19 suggests that, like Ebola survivors, some of them continue to experience long-term health consequences after recovering from their infections. With approximately 40% of all infected persons in West Africa dying from the Ebola virus during the 2014 epidemic, the West African case also represents the kind of high case-fatality event that we should be prepared to confront in future epidemics.[18]

Although there is no question that the Ebola epidemic was less global in its consequences compared to the COVID-19 pandemic, it was of particular significance because its most devastating consequences were observed in some of the world's poorest countries. These countries and their less-developed counterparts largely remain ill equipped to respond to future epidemics. Barring dramatic improvements in economic progress in these countries, they may once again need to prepare to confront the social consequences of an Ebola-like outbreak in the future—a task that would require building on the lessons learned from previous epidemics.

Survivors, Epidemics, and Society

Survivors of epidemics can facilitate progress on these issues because they are positioned to experience and observe the social transitions that occur after outbreaks of disease. However, developing new insights about these transitions can be complicated by the fact that the term "survivor" has several meanings. In its simplest form, the term describes those who are still alive after experiencing a potentially fatal event that takes the lives of others. When used in the context of epidemics, however, this phenomenon of remaining alive is important because it implies a return to normal health after being infected with a disease.

The survivors examined in this book fall into this general category of individuals. Like their counterparts who survived other epidemics, they represent a continuity of lived experiences that started before epidemics and continued after the end of these events. Survivors also embody the traumatic consequences of infectious diseases, which, although not always visible to the naked eye, continue to live on in their hearts and minds.[19] Other studies have attested to this by showing that such traumatic experiences of illnesses are difficult to forget. For example, survivors of the 1918 influenza epidemic often recalled their experiences with what they referred to as either the worse sickness they ever had, or experiences that left them so miserable that they did not care whether they survived.[20] As such, even though persons who were uninfected in their communities may forget the details of their own negative experiences, many of these details remain vivid in the minds of survivors and affect their everyday experiences.

Focusing on the experiences of individuals who recovered from Ebola virus infections is further important because it emphasizes what has been referred to as the "sufferer's role" in the history of healing.[21] This emphasis on survivors' experience is important because it recognizes the role of experiences, beliefs, and behaviors in shaping the lives of those who lived through the consequences of epidemics. The narratives they tell not only provide firsthand accounts of their experiences of trauma but also allow us to identify those who are most susceptible to the vulnerabilities associated with recovery. These vulnerabilities include susceptibility to opportunistic infections, limited access to social networks due to the mortality effects of Ebola among their close kin, and the problem of becoming fully accepted by members of their communities.

This does not discount the fact that Ebola survivors have other characteristics that distinguish them from the survivors of many recent epidemics. For one, they lived through an outbreak of a disease that was unfamiliar to them and for which there was no known cure. Widespread poverty in the countries where these outbreaks occurred suggests that the implications of the epidemic for the socioeconomically disadvantaged in West Africa are likely to be worse compared to those observed during, for example, the COVID-19 pandemic. Ebola survivors in West Africa include farmers in rural villages, the unemployed, and socially marginalized people living in urban slums. Many of them lived in greater levels of poverty than citizens in other countries. Partly as a result of their marginalized status, individuals from these lower socioeconomic groups accounted for most of the people infected during the epidemic.[22] To be clear, Ebola survivors also included people from higher socioeconomic groups, such as doctors, nurses, and other professionals. However, it remains unclear whether socioeconomic differences contributed to variations in the chances of survival from the disease. The two cases described at the start of the chapter, however, suggest that middle-class Ebola patients who were health care professionals were more likely than other patients to receive an early diagnosis and to be treated in modern health facilities. These variations could shape the social experiences of survivors if, for example, differential access to treatment created inequalities in the likelihood of experiencing the long-term health consequences of Ebola infection.

Regardless of socioeconomic status, Ebola survivors returning to their communities had other issues to confront, given the fact that these communities were themselves subject to the disruptive consequences of the epidemic. Therefore, the changes Ebola survivors experience in their post-epidemic life circumstances occur within communities that are also going through the process of social transformation. Evidence suggests that the economic fallout of epidemics within communities can have negative effects on the lives of survivors. Following the end of the plague epidemic in the Middle East in the fourteenth century, for example, the search for sustenance among survivors was made worse by the increases in the prices of food commodities as well as by decreases in salaries.[23] In the same vein, Ebola survivors returning to rural communities face similar constraints. In villages where communal farms need to be prepared for cultivation, survivors' contributions to the process could be limited by the lack of labor that would have been provided by family members lost to the disease. Such changes within communities and their impacts on survivors are among the least obvious transformations that shape overall well-being in the aftermath of epidemics.

These changes can be put into a useful perspective by improving what we know about the long-term health consequences of exposure to the Ebola virus infection. Health limitations can affect not only Ebola survivors' ability to participate in economic activity but also the degree to which they are involved in the social lives of their communities. Prior epidemics suggest that the health of survivors is rarely fully restored to what it was before the onset of disease. For example, survivors of smallpox epidemics have been found to face long-term vulnerabilities to bacterial infection, malnutrition, and loss of vision.[24,25] The health challenges observed after Ebola epidemics are similarly extensive and include lost vision, neurological problems, and musculoskeletal conditions. These conditions require some survivors to live with a loss of physical functionality and in need of medical attention for the rest of their lives.

By examining the diverse circumstances of Ebola survivors, the social transformations in their communities, and the various obstacles they face to social integration, this book hopes to provide a vivid assessment of how they have fared since the 2014 epidemic. Developing this portrait requires careful consideration of specific issues, such as an evaluation of the opportunities that survivors encounter after they recover. Moreover, it requires an investigation into whether ongoing processes of social change have either helped or hurt survivors' integration into their communities. Finally, it calls for an examination of the effectiveness of the available systems of social support that are supposed to help survivors deal with the various losses they have encountered.

Recovering from Epidemics

Determining how well societies have recovered from global epidemics can be challenging, because there is no consensus on what the process actually entails. Recovery does not simply occur as a result of the mere fact that an epidemic has ended. Instead, it is a process that is associated with a return to a prior status, and that process lasts from the end of an event to sometime in the future. Seen from the context of humanitarian disasters, recovery is sometimes used to describe the extended process of returning to pre-disaster norms.[26] This perspective underscores the expectation of returning to normal after experiencing unexpected societal disruptions. What is considered "normal" is itself very ambiguous. Too often, it is assumed that the goal of recovery is returning to a normal defined by the comparatively more favorable circumstances that existed before an epidemic. However, this goal only makes sense to the extent that things lost during these disruptions can truly be replaced.

Interest groups in societies emerging from epidemics have their own goals and assumptions about what recovery involves. For many government institutions, it involves eliminating the immediate threat to public health and restoring the main functions of their administrations. Survivors also have their own goals for recovery, which extend beyond the receipt of relief assistance. In some cases, governments and survivors disagree on which goals to prioritize. In Sierra Leone, for example, the government's central priorities after the end of the 2014 epidemic included restoring socioeconomic services and reversing economic growth rates that had declined.[27] However, Ebola survivors, believing that actions were being taken against their interests, sued the government to ensure that these interests were protected.[28] Moreover, as will be seen in the accounts provided by these survivors, the further away we move from the end of the epidemic, the more they believe that their government's actions have neither improved their circumstances nor helped to make them sufficiently independent.

Successful recovery from epidemics depends on other factors besides the responses of survivors. Variations in population size can possibly affect the duration of recovery and how well societies recover; other factors being equal, large populations expose more people to disease pathogens during epidemics than small populations. Added to this are the complications associated with differences in the lethality of specific threats to population health. Epidemics associated with viruses such as the bubonic plague are far more likely to be followed by challenging periods of recovery compared to those associated with, for example, the seasonal flu.

Some of the best examples of these influences were observed in previous centuries. For example, during the bubonic plague epidemic in Europe from 1348 to 1351, the continent lost between a third and half of its population and took several decades to recover from these demographic losses.[29] In comparison, the 1918 influenza epidemic killed about 18% of Europe's population in 6 weeks.[30] However, the population recovered within a decade as a result of increases in marriage and a rebound in childbearing. These examples, though, do not imply that the recovery of demographic indicators after epidemics is so simple. From 1518 to 1613, epidemics of smallpox and other diseases among Timucuan-speaking Native Americans reduced the size of their population by more than 50%. Since then, no evidence has been presented to show that their populations fully recovered.[31]

Other aspects of the recovery process can be affected by policy choices. Government policies can shape outcomes through the types of strategies they use to respond to the welfare of survivors. For example, following the end of the bubonic plague in Manchuria in China in the late 1900s, the government responded by making survivors members of the Chinese Communist Party after they were "liberated from their superstitious beliefs" about how to combat the spread of the disease.[32] More recent policy interventions have attempted to comprehensively target the instrumental needs of survivors. For example, NGOs sometimes attempt to help survivors by reducing the effects of post-traumatic stress disorders and providing income support, housing assistance, and other similar services. However, the lack of corresponding action to increase the sustainability of these interventions has limited NGOs' ability to fully support the long-term well-being of affected populations.

When recovery is effective, it should ideally lead to some sort of restoration of livelihoods. However, the extent to which this restoration process occurs has not been fully examined in societies recovering from Ebola epidemics. Studies on historical epidemics, however, indicate that some strategies used to accomplish this goal, such as the transfer of resources from the deceased to survivors, are not viable options. This is because new infections can be contracted by touching the belongings of the dead.[33] Other authors have downplayed these livelihood concerns by suggesting that the economic needs of survivors can be addressed by the reduced competition for resources (as a result of mortality), which follows the end of epidemics.[34] As observed after the Black Death in Europe during the 1300s, however, survivors are not always inclined to resume the exploitation of resources after the dust has settled.[35] As such, alternative sources of livelihoods need to be provided for them until they are able to fully participate in economic activity.

The Recovery of Survivors Following Ebola Epidemics

Evidence from the more than 20 Ebola epidemics that have occurred since 1976 provides some of the best examples of what follows after these outbreaks are over. To mark the end of these outbreaks, leaders usually begin by lauding the contributions of the various groups that worked together to control the spread of the disease. These are quintessentially cathartic moments that include a lot of celebration that reflects how seriously various actors took their mission to fight against the virus. At the end of the 1995 Ebola epidemic in Kikwit, Zaire, the WHO official who led the effort to contain the disease celebrated by saying, "We did it. We beat the virus."[36] After the last Ebola patient was released from hospital at the end of the 2020 Ebola epidemic in the Democratic Republic of the Congo, hospital staff similarly celebrated by dancing while drumming on trashcans.[37] As these celebrations subside, leading international organizations take time to acknowledge how strategies such as intensive social mobilization and behavior-specific advice helped to stop the spread of the disease.

What we know about how the affected communities themselves recover from Ebola epidemics generally comes from two sources. The first is research on primate populations. Until recent decades, few accounts were available of how human communities recovered from Ebola outbreaks because they mostly occurred in isolated rural settlements. Observations on the consequences of Ebola on ape and gorilla populations were thus used to fill these gaps and assess how rapidly primates can recover from these disasters. Interest in their recovery was partly driven by the fact that these primates are usually used as tourist attractions. As such, assessments of their welfare were motivated by the need to understand how well rural economies in the places where they lived recovered after the end of these Ebola outbreaks.[38]

The results of these assessments are largely intuitive. They confirm the high mortality impact of Ebola outbreaks on chimpanzee and gorilla populations while providing some of the first insights into the broader demographic consequences of the outbreaks. Following the 2004 Ebola outbreak among western lowland gorillas in Lokoué, Republic of Congo, for example, the population of solitary males increased during the recovery period because of higher levels of Ebola mortality among females than males.[39] The social consequences of these deaths were also among those one would expect to observe after high-mortality events. They included a decrease in the number of primates living in communal groups, increased instability within breeding groups, and a decline in migration between primate communities. The lower likelihood of migration was due to the fact that higher levels of Ebola mortality existed in traditional communities of out-migration compared to communities of in-migration.[40]

Observations from primate populations are now supplemented by information from a second source—namely, studies on the impacts of Ebola on human populations. Although the scale of Ebola infections in prior epidemics is limited compared to that observed during the 2014 West African epidemic, the insights provided by the former are instructive. A case in point is what was observed after the 2001 Ebola epidemic in Gulu, Uganda, which killed 425 people. During the recovery period, adults who were previously infected with disease continued to live with the long-term health consequences of the virus, including memory loss, blindness, and poor mental health.[41] Some of the evidence emerging from countries affected by the 2014 Ebola epidemic points to similar issues.

In terms of the social dimensions of recovery, most studies on human populations begin by confirming that the process of being infected is itself driven by the performance of various social roles. Accordingly, at the end of the 1995 Ebola epidemic in Kikwit, it was determined that almost all those who survived the outbreak became infected after caring for sick family members.[42] After returning to their communities, it was hard for them to reconcile their own willingness to care for others with the negative experiences they had while admitted to hospitals. Memories of these experiences, which included healthcare personnel refusing to provide care for them, were retained by survivors in the months following their recovery. Returning home also posed additional challenges as a result of the rejection they experienced from their friends, family members, and other members of their communities.[43] This rejection led to feelings of a loss of self-worth and altered their ability to perform many of the social roles they had performed in the past.

Compared to what we know about these outcomes, very little is known about how the economic circumstances of survivors are transformed after Ebola epidemics. However, recent evidence raises significant concern about their ability to return to their former sources of livelihood. Accordingly, approximately 90% of Ebola survivors in Guinea have experienced declines in their socioeconomic status,[44] while more than a third of their counterparts in Sierra Leone were unemployed after they recovered.[45] At the same time, observations made following the 2001 Ebola epidemic in Gulu indicate that Ebola survivors typically act to improve their own welfare. One of the most important actions survivors can take is to form a post-Ebola victims association tasked with helping survivors return to their normal lives and advocating for specialized forms of assistance.[46] These displays of agency were needed to fill the gap created by the lack of public investments to reverse the declines in survivors' well-being observed in the aftermath of the outbreak.

On the whole, much of what we have learned about the welfare of Ebola survivors in both primate and human populations is disconcerting. More concerning is the fact that the central mechanisms that explain these suboptimal social outcomes are not fully understood. Additionally, available evidence neither provides a basis for understanding how these limitations affect other aspects of the lives of survivors nor helps us understand the full range of alternatives available to survivors for improving these outcomes. Examining the experiences of survivors of the world's largest Ebola epidemic, however, can help us address these gaps in knowledge and provide new insights for developing appropriate interventions.

Meaning-Making Among Survivors of Epidemics

As central as these experiences are to our understanding, few things can help to put them in perspective as much as the ways in which they are interpreted by survivors themselves. Time provides an opportunity for them to reflect on the tragic events of the epidemics and use these reflections to evaluate their outlook on life. Meaning-making, as this process is called, underscores the importance of survivors as social individuals who live complex lives. Some of these complexities can be captured by an analysis of survivors' socioeconomic outcomes. However, meaning-making provides an added perspective by addressing how survivors use these experiences to adjust to the demands of their circumstances.

Leveraging the perspectives offered by meaning-making processes can allow us to identify multiple patterns of interpretation of these experiences. Two examples of these were observed following the 2001 Ebola epidemic in Gulu.[47] The first was characterized by interpretations of despondency and was more prevalent among survivors who saw themselves as victims. Their reflections on their experiences stirred up anxieties about the negative consequences of infection and increased concerns about whether their lives would ever return to normal. The second interpretation was more optimistic and was observed among those who had a positive outlook on their recovery. These survivors used their experiences with the virus as a source of inspiration to develop new goals for their lives.

This dual perspective provides a springboard for extending what we know about how meaning-making occurs at the end of Ebola epidemics. Whether it sufficiently captures the ways in which survivors come to terms with their experiences, though, is unclear. We do know, however, that the outcome of meaning-making processes can affect decisions made by people who had previously contracted the disease.

Survivors in West Africa who used meaning-making to develop a sense of optimism were more likely to be spurred into action, compared to those

who were more despondent. They increasingly participated in the donation of convalescent plasma to other Ebola patients, and subsequent research showed that these patients were less likely to die compared to their
counterparts who did not receive donated plasma.[48] Within treatment
centers, the more inspired survivors played active roles in the provision
of health care to infected patients. They were trained to become nursing
assistants who helped with basic tasks, such as the feeding of patients in
ETUs.[49] Because survivors had developed immunity to the disease, the risk
of them becoming reinfected with the virus was considerably low. As community members who spoke local languages, they were also seen as being
among the best candidates to work as translators for foreign medical workers communicating with patients.[50] Still others carved out broader roles in
advocacy and disease prevention in their post-epidemic communities as
a way of increasing public awareness of the lingering consequences of the
disease faced by their members.

While these outcomes are encouraging, there is still a lot we do not
know about these responses. Rarely is attention given to Ebola survivors with
more despondent interpretations of their experiences—to investigate their
respective action or lack of action to address the consequences of the epidemics. Additionally, we cannot assume that all meaning-making processes
fit into the clear dichotomies found in previous studies. Combinations of
these perspectives, if they exist, must be recognized and investigated to
determine their implications. We also cannot conclude that the actions
of survivors with more positive interpretations of their experiences are
limited to their participation in advocacy organizations. It is quite possible
that this ability to demonstrate agency and promote social change extends
to other areas of their lives. More importantly, it is important to recognize
that such actions are not taken in isolation but are themselves affected by
social, economic, and health constraints. Years after being diagnosed with
acute poliomyelitis, for example, people living with the disease made decisions about their professional trajectories based on the severity of their
symptoms.[51] Living with the chronic effects of prior Ebola infections may
have similar consequences for the life trajectories of survivors, and this
self-perception is important for understanding how they see themselves
within their communities.

Developing New Insights into the Social Dimensions of Epidemics

Shifting attention from the disruptions caused by epidemics to the factors that help societies recover from them offers new opportunities for expanding what we know about the challenges faced by Ebola survivors. This shift allows us to investigate how systems of inequality facilitate the creation of disparities in the outcomes survivors experience as they recover in their communities. Additionally, it allows us to identify deficits in their socioeconomic well-being that could be addressed to improve their experiences. Any new insight developed to understand the social dimensions of recovery should help provide answers to the question of how much progress Ebola survivors have made in their efforts to return to the lives they had before the epidemic. By attempting to meet this objective, the rest of the book addresses issues that further underscore the importance of the social dimensions of epidemics.

Chapter 2 contributes to the process by highlighting the pitfalls of official announcements made by organizations such as the WHO to mark the end of epidemics. In the case of the West African Ebola epidemic, the announcement was followed by the departure of most NGOs working in the affected countries, which helped to shift attention from the long-term consequences of the epidemic. The chapter then presents a conceptual basis for understanding why the social dimensions of recovery are important. While the components of these dimensions are diverse, the chapter argues that three of these are particularly important for evaluating the well-being of Ebola survivors. These dimensions are resilience, social structure, and the political economy of recovery. Together, they determine how individuals, systems of inequality, and institutions shape the kinds of outcomes we can expect to observe among Ebola survivors a decade after the end of the 2014 epidemic.

The first look into the accounts provided by survivors of their experiences in the aftermath of the epidemic is provided in chapter 3. The chapter traces Ebola survivors' journeys of recovery from ETUs to the mostly reconfigured households to which they returned. Based on their accounts, the chapter argues that, in part, robust social responses are warranted because of the dramatic changes that have occurred in the structure of affected families. The chapter specifically addresses the challenges faced by widows who must now provide for their children on their own, the welfare of orphans who are now homeless, and the plight of survivors abandoned by their spouses after they contracted the virus. Additionally, it discusses the challenges survivors face in rebuilding their families by forming new romantic relationships. These challenges are situated within the larger context of the new realities that now define the social lives of Ebola survivors.

Chapter 4 focuses on the long-term health consequences of Ebola infection, and how they continue to affect the well-being of many survivors. A central argument made in the chapter is that while the health complications of Ebola provide an opportunity for leveraging the benefits of both the medical and social responses to the epidemic, this opportunity has not been fully exploited. The chapter describes the wide range of morbidity outcomes that have been observed among Ebola survivors. Focusing on the social implications of these complications, it highlights the specific ways in which Ebola-related disabilities constrain the everyday experiences of survivors. The chapter also highlights how these disabilities affect survivors' ability to form social relationships, participate in community life, and return to work. Moreover, it describes the problems Ebola survivors continue to face in receiving access to health care. In particular, it argues that the social consequences of this lack of access to care include an increase in self-medication and the use of traditional African medicine, which, despite its advantages, has many limitations.

Focusing on social relationships between Ebola survivors and other community members, chapter 5 examines the lingering effects of stigma on the social well-being of survivors. Stigma, the chapter argues, continues to be encountered by survivors in family, job, and neighborhood contexts. Moreover, it continues to take a negative toll on the well-being of survivors. Part of this, the chapter argues, is due to the problematic strategy used in Ebola prevention campaigns of telling members of the public that Ebola has no cure. Consequently, many people still refuse to accept survivors who have fully recovered from the disease. While these challenges are apparent, however, institutional responses to them have been limited. Despite this problem, the chapter shows how survivors have developed their own social responses for navigating the effects of stigma to have meaningful social experiences in their communities.

Chapter 6 uses the economic consequences of Ebola virus infections to argue that many survivors have experienced declines in their socioeconomic circumstances since the end of the epidemic. These declines, it suggests, are due to at least three factors. The first is associated with disease-control protocols that called for the burning of the belongings of Ebola-infected persons during the epidemic, as well as the corresponding failure to replace the belongings that were destroyed. The second is the combined effect of the continued stigma and health limitations faced by many survivors, while the third is associated with problems in the distribution of humanitarian aid. While these problems have generally led to downward social mobility among Ebola survivors, many of them have found various ways to deal with these challenges and seek alternative sources of livelihood.

The final chapter ends by making the case for an equal level of attention to be given to the medical and social consequences of epidemics. It argues that an increased emphasis on social responses is especially needed in developing countries emerging from epidemics. Affected populations in these regions include socially marginalized people who were already living in poverty before the start of epidemics. The chapter emphasizes the need for investments in both the medical and social consequences of epidemics to mimic the two-pronged approach used to address the diverse consequences of the COVID-19 pandemic. At the same time, the chapter describes how the experiences of Ebola survivors differ from those of survivors of the pandemic. Finally, the chapter discusses the lessons learned from the experiences of Ebola survivors and possible ways in which the importance of social issues can be elevated in the development of policy.

2 Social Determinants of Recovery

Oﬃcial announcements about the end of epidemics usually give limited attention to the challenges that lie ahead. When the WHO announced the end of Liberia's Ebola outbreak on June 6, 2016, things were not that different.[1] The announcement began by noting that no new case of the disease had been recorded for 42 days since the last infected person tested negative for the virus twice. Thereafter, the announcement described what the WHO would focus on in the weeks ahead. The following 90 days, it noted, would be a period of heightened surveillance to ensure that any new cases of Ebola would be identified quickly.[2] Subsequently, it intended to ensure that survivors had the resources they needed to be reintegrated into their communities. A vital aspect of the organization's long-term focus was also identified. This involved the WHO's plan to work with its partners to develop a resilient health system in Liberia during the post-epidemic period. There is no question that these priorities were appropriate. No one would dispute the importance of improving health care delivery systems in the countries affected by the epidemic. Nor would anyone question the need to assist Ebola survivors in returning to their communities.

About a decade after these priorities were announced, however, it has become clear that they are yet to have the positive impact they were expected to have on the lives of Ebola survivors. Yet, this is one reason why recovery from epidemics is far more complicated than what official announcements suggest. Recovery does not happen simply because we plan for it. Instead, it is an extensive process that occurs in specific social contexts. Ideally, it should address the challenges encountered by the survivors while at the same time increasing investments in their institutions, such as their families and voluntary organizations. When it becomes clear that the challenges of survivors are continuing, questions must be asked to determine why this is the case and what the challenges imply for their everyday experiences. Studying the lives of survivors of epidemics provides one way of answering these questions while developing a comprehensive perspective on the social dimensions of life after epidemics.

The social factors that influence processes of recovery are diverse. However, a few of them are particularly important for assessing how well these processes progress. The first set of factors that determine how recovery occurs includes those associated with individual experiences. These are experiences observed among individuals such as Ebola survivors. They are affected by factors such as their health status, which determines their ability to return to their pre-epidemic activities, and their level of education, which influences their access to resources. Apart from these, individual experiences are also affected by the new challenges faced by those who are unable to return to their normal lives as a result of their economic and social losses.

Social contexts provide a second set of factors that affect the success of recovery efforts, although their influence is less intuitive. This is because some of the effects of contexts are rooted in the pre-pandemic histories of communities emerging from crises. Characteristics of social contexts can further act to trigger humanitarian emergencies or accentuate their negative consequences. For example, refugee movements, ethnic conflicts, and civil unrest are sometimes driven by contextual characteristics such as class tensions, ancestral histories, and systems of inequality. Not surprisingly, such contextual characteristics were among the major determinants of the spread of the Ebola virus across West Africa after the initial outbreak in Guinea. Previous studies have shown, for example, that after the first case was observed in Meliandou, Guinea, the spread of the virus accelerated when it reached the Kissi-speaking groups in the tri-border region of Liberia, Guinea, and Sierra Leone.[3] These groups have ancestral connections that predate the start of the colonial period and continue to maintain these connections by moving freely across the borders of these countries.

Other characteristics of social contexts, such as social structure, determine the groups most likely to be exposed to the long-term consequences of epidemics. We now know, for instance, that epidemics do not have the same consequences among the various groups found in the places where they occur.[4] As such, given the fact that the most brutal consequences of the West African Ebola epidemic were observed among some of the poorest and most marginalized populations in the region,[5] we can expect these groups to face some of the most daunting difficulties in their recovery from the disease.

Contextual factors are so embedded in the fabric of communities that their influence on the course of epidemics is difficult to ignore. Moreover, because many of their effects are enduring, they persist even after official declarations are made to mark the end of epidemics. During the recovery process, contextual factors can determine which house is repaired and which is not. They can also affect who gets access to humanitarian relief and who does not. They even determine which groups are officially designated as victims of epidemics, which can control access to a wide range of resources. Moreover, they can affect how well institutions, interest groups, and affected communities participate in the recovery process themselves.

Apart from the influence of contextual factors, the recovery of communities is also shaped by the forces that operate beyond their borders. These macro-level factors include political systems, economic institutions, and the role of the global actors who make decisions about how to respond to epidemics. Also considered to be among a broad range of political economy influences, these factors can explain how the failure to develop strong national institutions affects to what extent societies can withstand the shocks created by epidemics. They further explain how decisions are made about the allocation of resources, why traditions of accountability are underdeveloped, and why some societies depend on foreign relief assistance after epidemics more than others do.

All told, a significant diversity of factors determine what we should expect to observe while societies recover from the disruptions caused by these crises. However, it is important to limit our understanding of these influences to a core set of factors that determine the success of the recovery efforts of the West African communities that were affected by the epidemic. Accomplishing this objective requires answers to one crucial question: What are the major social factors that explain how well Ebola survivors are able to adjust to the demands of life after the end of the epidemic?

Three perspectives are used to answer this question. The first comes from studies on resilience, which highlight how individual-level factors affect responses to crises. The second is based on the sociology of disasters and emphasizes how contextual factors, such as social structure, determine the welfare of survivors. The third emphasizes the importance of macro-level factors, focusing specifically on the political economy of societies recovering from epidemics. Together, these perspectives provide a useful start for assessing the progress made so far in the social integration of Ebola survivors into their communities.

Resilience and Recovery

Resilience is widely used to describe how individuals, communities, and institutions recover from crises. However, the most commonly used application of the concept is found in the analysis of individual experiences. This does not mean that these experiences exist in isolation. In fact, the interdependence between these experiences and other factors is recognized in studies on social resilience, which capture how individuals and groups develop social relationships after experiencing adversity.[6] Among individuals, however, resilience can be considered as an outcome determined by the collective resources available to individuals to facilitate their recovery. The origin of the concept itself is unclear. However, it has long been used to capture the human fascination with how individuals rebound after experiencing harmful events. This explains why ideas about resilience have been found across millennia and societies in ancient legends about overcoming adversity.[7]

Applications of the concept of resilience to understand individual experiences usually focus on positive adaptations to life as people recover from adverse experiences. This understanding of the process of recovery can be seen from multiple perspectives.[8] One of these is related to observations of better-than-expected outcomes among high-risk individuals who experienced adversity. Another is used to understand how individuals regain effective or normal functioning following conditions of overwhelming adversity, while a third is used for understanding how effective functioning is maintained under very adverse conditions.

Each of these perspectives has been used to examine how infected persons fared during the Ebola crisis. For example, a key question medical professionals tried to answer during the 2014 epidemic was why some infected individuals had better-than-expected outcomes compared to others.

At that time, it was easy to assume that, at least in terms of medical outcomes, those who had the best outcomes were individuals who were diagnosed quite early and were thus likely to receive treatment sooner. Concerns have also been expressed about the problems Ebola survivors face while trying to regain their normal functions after they are released from ETUs.[9] These concerns have informed several studies that seek to assess how well survivors are able to regain their physical health. Less attention has been given to assessing their ability to maintain effective functions under adverse conditions.

Perhaps this is because many previous studies on Ebola survivors are not designed to determine whether the challenges they experience are temporary or permanent. In some cases, the evidence has implied that these challenges are short-term hardships. For example, approximately 1 year after the start of the 2014 epidemic, a study of 25 Ebola survivors argued that they had 2 sources of resilience that helped them bounce back from illness.[10] These were identified as self- or community preservation and coping resources such as their faith in God. While there is no question that these sources are important, the study could not determine whether these sources continued to be important as survivors attempted to integrate into their community in the years that followed.

Part of the problem of understanding these long-term implications stems from the fact that scholarly interest in epidemics significantly declines after they are over. As a result, the tendency to use short-term perspectives to examine the resilience of survivors extends beyond studies on Ebola. Following the 2002 SARS epidemic, for example, an attempt to was made to identify differences in the ability of infected persons to recover after they were hospitalized. Individuals who were considered more resilient were those able to regain their physical health much faster than those who were not, and the outcomes of the former were attributed to their access to high levels of social support.[11] However, recovery from illness is not a process that ends after patients are released from hospitals. As such, attention needs to be given to the health outcomes of survivors during the extended stages of recovery.

Care must, however, be taken to avoid trivializing the significance of short-term perspectives on the role of resilience. Indeed, these perspectives are particularly useful for developing portraits of the welfare of survivors at specific points in time. For example, their focus on recovery from illnesses after survivors are discharged from hospitals is important for illuminating what happens at the start of their long journeys of recovery. Restricting ourselves to short-term understandings of resilience, however, risks minimizing the complexities faced by survivors as they work toward the state of well-being they had before they were infected. Short-term perspectives cannot fully capture these complexities, since a return to a former state of wellbeing is not always a short-term process.

Additionally, for many Ebola survivors, a return to normal health functioning is simply not an option. Permanent disabilities and irreversible health complications require them to adjust their lives around these new realities. The new normal, which defines their experiences, introduces new challenges, demands new responses, and requires a nuanced understanding of resilience. Many of these permanent health challenges faced by Ebola survivors do not fit neatly into existing frameworks of resilience. As such, extended applications of the concept of resilience are needed to capture their current realities.

The argument for using new or related perspectives for understanding individual experiences of recovery is not necessarily novel. This approach has been discussed in studies examining the realities faced by people with HIV/AIDS. As more people live with the disease longer than was possible in previous decades, scholars have increased their attempts to understand how alternative perspectives of resilience can be used to examine everyday experiences. One of these alternatives is the use of the concept of hardiness. Unlike traditional notions of resilience, hardiness describes the ability to thrive over the long term while living with health limitations. The term further captures a sense of meaningfulness and purpose in life, a sense of control, and a realization that change can provide an opportunity for growth.[12] More importantly, hardiness is associated with long-term adaptations to harsh conditions and the ability to respond to the unending difficulties individuals encounter in their daily activities. Hardiness, therefore, implies a high level of persistence that is considered to be a critical factor that helps individuals become resilient in their response to stressful events.[13]

Another limitation of short-term perspectives on resilience is that they can affect the longevity of actions taken to improve the well-being of survivors. Development experts now see this as a serious problem. They argue that, to most international development agencies, resilience is nothing more than a buzzword that reinforces the status quo, ignores the vulnerability of individuals, and reduces the prospect of achieving true transformation.[14] One consequence of this is that development agencies are more comfortable designing interventions that provide short-term relief after periods of crises than creating strategies that address the long-term needs of individuals. The former strategy is limiting, while the latter focuses on building resilience for the long haul. Focusing on this long-term perspective requires development agencies to be continuously engaged with affected communities, make long-term commitments, and conduct an extensive analysis of contexts.[15] This approach is effective because it links the response to an immediate crisis to an extended intervention strategy—that is, one that, among other things, makes investments in individuals to improve their livelihoods and their access to resources in their communities.

Unfortunately, this more extended strategy has not been fully adopted in recovering communities in West Africa in the years following the 2014 Ebola epidemic. Instead, much of what has been observed is inconsistent with this need for long-term engagement with Ebola survivors to prepare them for the long haul. While concerns about the global threat of Ebola led to one of the most significant responses of international aid agencies to a crisis in the region, the rapid departure of NGOs after the epidemic was a lost opportunity to build on these responses and make their impacts sustainable. In the absence of a sustained strategy for building resilience, the rapid end of the work of these agencies has left serious gaps in the provision of essential services. As a result, aid agencies have missed important opportunities for linking relief aid to development.

Social Structure and Recovery

Social contexts help to determine the conditions under which recovery occurs. However, few characteristics of these contexts are as important for shaping the process as much as those associated with social structure. Considered to include the roles, arrangements, relationships, and institutions found within societies, social structure provides the central basis for how communities operate. It determines interactions between groups, social norms, and social responsibilities. Moreover, it is important for providing some form of predictability in social relations within communities.

Therefore, when recovery efforts focus on medical needs without giving equal consideration to social structure, they ignore a critical factor that determines the extent to which recovery can truly occur.

Some of the earliest efforts to acknowledge the significance of social structure for the recovery of communities were done by scholars in the field of political ecology. These scholars argue that the physical conditions of communities are less important determinants of what occurs after humanitarian disasters than the social conditions in these communities. A central basis for this argument is that characteristics such as social structure can create continuities and discontinuities in progress toward recovery as well as new vulnerabilities in the post-disaster environments of communities.[16]

Most of the arrangements that define the social structure of communities are usually established before the start of epidemics. However, the disruptions caused by these events can negatively affect key elements of these arrangements. For example, the disruptions can lead to declines in the social position of women, increased class tensions, and changes in the configuration of households. Some of these disruptions have been observed in the aftermath of the Ebola epidemic. In both Liberia and Sierra Leone, for example, the epidemic was followed by increases in gender-based violence against girls and young women and high rates of teen pregnancy, even among those who were not infected by the virus.[17] Other epidemics have also been followed by disruptions in household structure and the reorganization of relationships between families.

Such changes tend to be particularly prevalent after epidemics with high levels of mortality. For instance, during the Great Plague of London in 1665, a large number of women died during childbirth due to the lack of midwives, resulting in an increase in the number of widowers.[18] Similarly, after the flu epidemic of 1918, which led to higher levels of mortality among children and young mothers,[19] social recovery occurred in contexts defined by decreases in family sizes and increases in the number of orphans. These changes in family configuration can have other social consequences. One of these is the disruption of financial arrangements due to the loss of income earners, which can lead to a reorganization of the relationships between households and their communities.

For persons who survive epidemics after being infected, disruptions can also lead to a reconfiguration of social structure and the loss of social values due to the lingering stigma of disease.[20] Driven by fear and the need to blame others, stigma is often used to reduce social interaction with those considered to be tainted. In the process, it can negatively affect the social arrangements and norms of social trust that existed before the start of epidemics. In Sierra Leone, for example, the stigma of Ebola resulted in shifts in social norms of trust, how people treated the sick, and how Ebola patients were treated after they were discharged from hospitals.[21]

Although systematic research on the long-term effects of these stigmas is limited, evidence indicates that they continue to linger in the communities that Ebola survivors returned to.[22] When stigma is deployed, the ostracization of the stigmatized undermines social values and can lead to a loss of social position.[23] This loss can have downstream effects on social relationships and standards of living, as reflected in studies showing an association between stigma and the loss of employment as well as social standing among people affected by HIV/AIDS.[24]

Notwithstanding the consequences of these disruptions, most other elements of social structure remain unaffected during epidemics and continue to influence how recovery processes unfold. Part of this influence is driven by the effects of vulnerability—a key factor that creates differential patterns of risk among individuals and places.[25] These differential risks can create new inequalities as the vulnerable become increasingly vulnerable and individuals on the margins of society become increasingly disadvantaged.

Some of these differential risk patterns occur when poor countries find it more difficult than their wealthier counterparts to recover from similar kinds of disasters. The most recent example of this was observed during the early phase of the COVID-19 pandemic, when countries such as Brazil recovered less rapidly from the worst consequences of the pandemic compared to wealthier countries such as the United States. Global patterns of vulnerability can similarly produce inequalities in individual outcomes of recovery from epidemics. During the 2014 Ebola epidemic, this was observed when almost every citizen of Western countries who was infected with the virus recovered from these infections, while most Africans who were similarly infected died from the disease.

Social structure can similarly be associated with unequal patterns of vulnerability in local communities, which can be exacerbated in the aftermath of epidemics. These unequal patterns are usually linked with indicators of disadvantage such as racial and gender minority status. Today, these factors shape social inequalities before the onset of epidemics as much as they increase the susceptibility of the disadvantaged to the consequences of these outbreaks.[26]

Existing studies provide many examples of epidemics that had more negative consequences for the socially marginalized than others in their societies. Some of these were observed during epidemics in the United States. Chinese immigrants in San Francisco, for example, faced multiple disadvantages during the bubonic plague of 1916. They not only had high rates of mortality from the disease but also had property destroyed by mobs blaming them for the spread of the disease,[27] which affected their recovery from the outbreak. Poor Jewish immigrants from Russia, who were similarly blamed for New York's typhoid fever epidemic in 1892, were also left worse off at the end of the epidemic than at the beginning.[28] Added to this, the negative consequences of the COVID-19 pandemic were generally concentrated among racial minority groups. As expected, research suggests that these groups now face some of the most significant obstacles to recovery compared to other groups in the United States.[29]

Social structure is therefore likely to be among the most important determinants of the unequal burden of recovery observed in West African communities affected by the 2014 Ebola epidemic.[30] In most African countries, the main elements of social structure that affect inequalities in well-being include factors such as ethnicity and region of origin. During the Ebola epidemic, however, the significance of these factors declined. Instead, the dimensions of social structure that contributed most to social inequalities were those associated with place of residence, that is, rural versus urban areas, and social class.[31]

Rural-urban disparities in Africa are more than just inequalities driven by geographical variations. They reflect differences in histories, opportunities for advancement, and the organization of communities. Rural-urban disparities are among the most enduring features of the social structure of many African countries. They originated in the pre-colonial period when traditional rulers such as kings and chiefs concentrated their administrative power and resources in larger settlements, which served as centers of power and authority, rather than in smaller villages.[32]

In the late 1800s, the disparity between urban and rural areas increased when colonial administrations took steps to increase development in the former at the expense of the latter. In Sierra Leone, for example, British investment in public infrastructure was heavily focused on the capital city, Freetown, and provincial headquarter towns, where colonial officers resided. Similar urban biases were observed in Liberia during this period, although the country did not have a formal colonial experience. Accordingly, since the late 1800s, Monrovia, the capital city, has received higher levels of government attention to the development of the health sector than rural areas. Whatever little investment was made in the health sector in rural areas was designed to target areas where cash crops such as rubber were produced.[33]

By the 1960s, the social organization of Liberian and Sierra Leonean societies had become increasingly defined by a symbiotic relationship between urban and rural areas. Two decades later, structural adjustment policies required by the International Monetary Fund in the two countries made things worse. Among other things, they required the elimination of government subsidies in the health care sector and the imposition of user fees to cover the costs of treatment. As a result, these policies led to significant increases in the health care costs of poor rural residents, who were paying more out of pocket as a percentage of household expenditure than wealthier households.[34]

Urban-rural inequalities are important for understanding other aspects of the social organization of both countries. In particular, these inequalities have fueled massive migrations from rural to urban areas, as rural residents migrated to city centers in search of better opportunities. As a result of these migrations, dramatic increases have occurred in the number of residents in these cities in recent decades. Between the 1960s and 2015, for example, Monrovia saw a tenfold increase in the size of its population,[35] while the corresponding increase in Freetown was approximately sevenfold.[36] In both cases, this growth has been accompanied by the expansion of slum settlements where arriving migrants and other marginalized groups live in high levels of poverty.

Slum residents now form a new underclass in these cities and are among the most socially marginalized groups. They lack access to essential services such as water supply, electricity, and health care and have less favorable outcomes than other urban residents in almost every indicator of social well-being. In Sierra Leone, members of this marginalized urban poor population have been referred to as part of the lumpen proletariat,[37] a permanent reservoir of lower-class individuals from whom politicians recruit people to foment violence. Correspondingly, their counterparts in urban Liberia have been described by one commentator as "gangsters who steal car batteries, rob people, and deal in drugs."[38] Given the lack of access to social and infrastructure services in slum settlements, it was not surprising that some of the most devastating consequences of the Ebola epidemic were observed in these communities. However, at the end of the epidemic, Ebola survivors who returned to these communities went back to living in the same squalid conditions that made them vulnerable to various social disruptions during the previous decades.

The fact that urban slum residents were vulnerable to the spread of Ebola should not distract from the reality that residents of rural areas were even more susceptible. In fact, before 2014, all major outbreaks of Ebola occurred in rural areas. The 2014 epidemic originated in rural Guinea, among people in one of the country's most marginalized communities. From there, it spread to Liberia and Sierra Leone through rural transport networks before it reached urban areas.[39] Coupled with the fact that rural areas are closer to forests, where the zoonotic transfer of the virus to humans most likely occurred, their marginalization from centers of power made it difficult to control the early spread of the virus. As a result, rural residents experienced many of the most deleterious consequences of the epidemic, which was made worse by their lack of access to functional health care facilities and the means to travel to these facilities.

These realities were captured in a Liberian assessment of rural counties affected by Ebola conducted by the US Centers for Disease Control and Prevention (CDC) and the country's government. The evaluation found that the four counties most affected by the epidemic could not control the outbreak because they lacked training and supplies, had limited access to roads, and had poor communications networks.[40] Two of these rural counties had no functioning ambulance. Additionally, only one lab technician was trained to handle blood samples from Ebola cases in all four counties. Moreover, health care workers in these counties lacked adequate access to personal protective equipment.

Despite the comparative marginalization of rural areas, the brunt of the consequences of marginalization in these areas during and after epidemics is faced by their even more disadvantaged residents. When people lack access to health infrastructure, the process of seeking health care places a higher burden on the poor than on the non-poor. Among poor villages near the Gola Forest around the border Liberia shares with Sierra Leone, travel to the nearest health center during the Ebola epidemic took between two hours and a full day. The actual duration depended on whether one could pay laborers to carry infected persons with a hammock.[41] Access to care in these areas has still not improved since the end of the epidemic.[42] Consequently, rural health centers are not equipped to serve the needs of Ebola survivors, which makes it difficult for these survivors to manage the health complications they continue to experience.

A final perspective on the significance of social structure can be provided by an examination of the activities of international relief organizations. Following the end of humanitarian emergencies, social structure is among the main factors that determine the effectiveness of their programs. Because social structure is so embedded in the social organization of communities, it can affect the provision of relief in ways that continue to reinforce existing systems of disadvantage. Social hierarchies can also make it difficult for socially marginalized groups to access resources from these programs because rules of eligibility and procedures of access are sometimes too cumbersome.[43] Apart from these barriers, relief programs can inadvertently reinforce social inequalities when they unduly focus on helping victims return to their pre-disaster conditions. This strategy can be limiting. For slum residents, it implies a return to living in slum conditions, while for rural residents, it implies a return to social marginalization. In some cases, communities can also be so devastated by epidemics that a return to pre-epidemic conditions is not a viable option. Many Ebola survivors find themselves in similar circumstances, which can preclude their return to the lives they had before. Their family members who died cannot be replaced, while some of the health complications they face cannot be reversed. These issues present long-term problems that relief programs are not designed to address. As a result, they are likely to lead to the downward social mobility of many Ebola survivors.

The Political Economy of Recovery

Political economy factors represent a final set of determinants of how well societies recover from epidemics. Operating at both the national and international levels, these factors can affect the social contexts of communities where recovery occurs and the trajectory of individual experiences of recovery. At the start of the 2014 Ebola epidemic, there was extensive interest in how political economy factors affected the crisis. The significance of these factors was seen as operating through the impacts of colonial legacies, structural adjustment programs, and foreign aid dependence, which combined to limit how well West African states could respond to the epidemic.[44] Most of these factors continue to affect the responses used to address the process of recovery.

As with social contexts, the role of political economy factors precedes the start of epidemics. Most of the structures of power, systems of accountability, macroeconomic vulnerabilities, and international relations that affect these responses were already in place before the index case of Ebola was observed. After epidemics begin, these influences can act to either accentuate or ameliorate the social disruptions in affected communities.

In the case of the Ebola epidemic, they made things worse. For one, the failure of governments to make the necessary investments in their health systems helped to transform what should have been a localized outbreak in Meliandou into the world's largest Ebola epidemic. Similarly, the WHO waited seven months before declaring the outbreak an international health emergency.[45] These failures made it difficult to mobilize the resources needed to control the spread of the virus. In fact, one can argue that the inaction of these institutions made them poorly prepared to address the initial spread of Ebola, which is partly responsible for the deplorable circumstances now faced by many survivors.

One useful strategy to think about the importance of political economy factors for periods of recovery is to consider them part of the dynamics of social relations. Studies on social relations build on the foundations developed by research on social structure to more broadly incorporate the role of institutions, power relations, and structures of dependence.[46] One study on the response to the Ebola epidemic in the slums of Sierra Leone has highlighted the influence of these factors. The authors argued that the response was inadequate because it neglected social relations in these communities by treating infected individuals while ignoring the poverty and social hierarchies that made these communities exist.[47] Given its focus on structures of dependence and social hierarchies, political economy analysis of recovery from epidemics requires an understanding of who controls whom, the relationships between governments and their citizens, and how these relationships affect access to resources.[48]

Political economy influences further include the role of global ideologies in shaping these relationships and the process of developing international responses to major problems. This process is observed when the hegemonic global model supported by international institutions is used to unduly focus on emergency responses to epidemics. Although this strategy is important in itself, it can distract from the need to make complementary social investments in vulnerable communities. Most of these agencies ignore this approach when making decisions on the allocation of resources to address the consequences of epidemics. In the process, more resources are allocated to implement short-term emergency responses, leaving fewer available for building the capacity of communities to sustain themselves in the long term.

Within states, political economy factors affect recovery processes in ways that are equally consequential. Countries with traditions of developing consensus on issues related to the welfare of their citizens are better able to marshal the resources needed to tackle the consequences of epidemics, compared to those without similar traditions. Such traditions of consensus building, coalition development, and government provision of the infrastructure needed to foster recovery are absent in many countries.[49] Moreover, the breakdown of these traditions and social relations between a government and its citizens can have devastating consequences that can limit a state's capacity to respond to health emergencies.

These consequences were observed in Liberia when the capacity of public institutions to prepare for such emergencies was eroded during the country's civil war that started in 1989. The war destroyed much of Liberia's physical and social infrastructure while weakening the effectiveness of institutions such as the hospitals and schools used to train health care professionals. Two years after the start of the civil war, rebels allied to Charles Taylor, leader of Liberia's most powerful rebel faction, started a civil war in neighboring Sierra Leone. This war had similar effects on the destruction of institutions. When the Ebola epidemic started about a decade after the end of both conflicts, Liberia and Sierra Leone were still in the process of rebuilding the institutions and systems that had been destroyed during these conflicts. Things have not improved in the years after the end of the epidemic. As a result of the economic losses experienced during this period, national revenues remained low in the years immediately following the end of the crisis, which limited the amount of investment that could be made to support the lives of Ebola survivors.[50]

Related to their role in determining the effectiveness of national institutions, political economy factors affect the development of national traditions of transparency and accountability. When such traditions are lacking, humanitarian disasters can be used to increase revenue, accrue personal wealth, or redistribute power through the allocation of more relief funds to political allies and fewer to the politically disconnected.[51] Some governments have even been known to underinvest in the prevention of humanitarian disasters because they expect international organizations to provide humanitarian relief when these disasters occur. Otherwise known as the racket effect,[52] this irresponsible display of leadership describes the tendency of governments to ignore the welfare of their citizens to attract international aid that could be used to increase personal wealth.

Political corruption can significantly affect recovery efforts in other important ways. Since Sierra Leone's independence in 1962, the use of state resources for personal gain has been an almost consistent feature of the country's political economy. As such, the state's ability to provide public goods and invest in its health care system has significantly declined.[53] The problem affects more countries than just Sierra Leone. A recent review of corruption in anglophone countries in West Africa, including Liberia, Nigeria, and Ghana, found various types of corrupt practices in their respective health care systems. These practices included bribery, the theft of drugs and supplies, and the diversion of patients from public to private hospitals.[54] The review specifically indicated that in Liberia, corruption increased public distrust of the health care system to such as extent that it became a major obstacle to controlling the spread of Ebola.[55] Similarly, in the three West African countries most affected by the epidemic, the disbursement of aid to affected communities was plagued by corruption and the diversion of relief funds for personal use.[56] As will be seen in the accounts provided by Ebola survivors, this does not mean that no government officials are committed to meeting the needs of the afflicted. However, it does mean that corruption has robbed survivors of the opportunity to begin their recovery on sound footing, which has had broader implications for their successful integration into their communities.

Shaping the Course of Ebola Recovery

Recovery from epidemics does not end with the departure of international relief agencies after the last infected person has been discharged. True recovery is an extended process that requires the rebuilding of all affected sectors in a society and investing in the lives of survivors. The latter is of particular significance because it is a social process often forgotten after the global media's attention turns elsewhere. Understanding the pathways to recovery taken by survivors requires an appreciation of the connections that exist between their own experiences and larger factors that operate in their communities.

As described above, the importance of this process can by understood by examining the multidimensional factors that help to make recovery successful. This starts with an appreciation of the importance of individual experiences, which help to explain how well survivors fare as they navigate the process of returning to what is left of their lives. Additionally, it involves recognizing that survivors live in social contexts that are strongly influenced by social structure. Finally, it requires that attention be given to the political economy of the response to the consequences of epidemics. This attention is needed not only to better understand international and national responses to epidemics but also to evaluate whether these responses are making a positive difference in the lives of Ebola survivors.

3 Family Life in the Aftermath of Ebola

Sometime around 2015, while Jernora's family lived in Monrovia, her husband decided to take care of his sick friend after learning that he was ill. Her family did not object; after all, such expressions of care were common in their community. When the men arrived at the John F. Kennedy Hospital in Monrovia, the patient was diagnosed as being infected with Ebola. Refusing to accept the diagnosis, they traveled to Lofa County, more than 100 miles away, to seek alternative medical treatments. Their quest was unsuccessful, and the friend died from the disease. Afterward, Jernora's husband returned to Monrovia and immediately started feeling ill. All 12 residents of the household were subsequently diagnosed with Ebola, including members of Jernora's immediate and extended families. As the number of infected persons increased, so did the number of deaths in the household. The first person to die was Jernora's husband. His death was followed by those of the couple's three children, her mother-in-law, and her sister-in-law. By the time the dust settled, 11 of the 12 infected persons had died of the disease, leaving Jernora as the only survivor.

Life as a survivor in families ravaged by Ebola usually begins as patients recover while they are still in ETUs. For Jernora, this involved managing the mixed emotions she experienced while she fought for her survival. On the one hand, she feared the possibility of dying, but on the other hand, she was mourning the loss of her loved ones. Recovering from the disease brought on a new set of challenges, most of which involved beginning her life as a widow. For one, she had no relatives of her own in Monrovia. She was not from the city and had been brought there by her husband after their marriage. Her main support system in Monrovia consisted of her in-laws, but this had been weakened by the Ebola deaths in their household.

With the loss of resources that followed the death of her husband, living as a widow had put her in objectively worse circumstances compared to those she had before her family was struck by Ebola.

Such changes in the dynamics of families were among the most consequential impacts of the 2014 Ebola epidemic in West Africa. While the types of family structures found in these contexts are diverse, Ebola deaths led to a reconfiguration of families that placed survivors in circumstances that made them more vulnerable than they were before. Some of them transitioned into new families where they lived as single parents caring for their surviving children. Others lived in families as parents who recovered from Ebola but lost their children to the disease. By far the most significant of these transitions were those that involved Ebola orphans, many of whom have struggled to manage the realities of daily life without the help of their parents.

While these transitions are important, putting an exclusive focus on them risks minimizing the scale of the devastation that occurred within families. It shifts attention away from complex mortality patterns that occurred within families, which have created new burdens for survivors as they recover from the crisis. These complexities are captured in the experiences of women like Jernora, who are not just widows who lost their spouses. Along with the experience of widowhood, they also deal with the stress of being mothers who lost their children and individuals who lost other relatives who lived in their households. Most Ebola orphans are distinguished from other orphans by their experience with these complex mortality losses. Unlike traditional orphans who are defined by the deaths of their parents, Ebola orphans lost parents as well as aunts, uncles, grandparents, and other relatives who could have stepped in to care for them.

The experience of confronting these consequences does not occur in isolation, because Ebola survivors have other issues to address as they adjust to their new familial circumstances. These include adapting to the loss of the emotional support, income, and other resources previously provided by their kin, who are now deceased. Surviving the epidemic can also lead to changes in the relationships between survivors and their extended family members who are still alive. For those who lost their spouses, recovery may further require a re-entry into the family formation processes of dating and marriage. All of these adjustments must occur while survivors navigate the personal health, psychological, and social changes that accompany recovery from a serious disease.

Given that families are considered to be among the most important social institutions,[1] it is important to examine the changes that occurred in their dynamics in the aftermath of the Ebola epidemic. How well survivors have adapted to these changes can determine the success of their recovery efforts, their adjustment to new types of family configurations, and the capacity of these configurations to meet their diverse needs. Addressing these issues requires that answers be provided to several questions. To what extent did Ebola deaths result in changes in the composition of families? How did the fragmentation of families due to these deaths affect how well survivors adjusted to life after returning to their communities? What constraints did survivors face in their efforts to start new families? Finally, have the disruptions to families caused by the epidemic led to notable changes in the material circumstances of survivors?

Norms, Crises, and the Dynamics of African Families

Families have long been at the center of the organization of social life in sub-Saharan Africa. Nevertheless, local perspectives on what constitutes a family in countries such as Liberia and Sierra Leone differ from Western notions of how families are defined. Farmer describes the view of how families are defined in Sierra Leone by noting that they can include a range of unrelated individuals. Older adults can be introduced as mothers and fathers, siblings do not always share the same parent, and uncles are sometimes just older cousins.[2] This diversity in definitions of what constitutes a family has also been documented in Liberia, reflecting the fluidity in the ways in which family relationships are understood in both countries.[3]

In terms of structure, families in both countries take on diverse forms depending on ethnicity, religion, and place of residence. Despite this variation, several common features exist in the norms surrounding how families function. For example, marriage is generally defined by traditional customs, especially in rural areas, and is contracted through social transactions such as the payment of a bride price or the performance of bride service.[4] Some scholars have argued that these practices have several advantages, one of which is that they make marriage to adults accessible regardless of social status. However, they have disadvantages as well, the most significant of which is the fact that the dissolution of these marriages can have more negative consequences for mothers and their children than for fathers.[5] Compared to their rural counterparts, urban residents in large cities such as Monrovia and Freetown are more likely to participate in statutory, Western-type marriages. However, the growing arrival of rural migrants in these cities has led to an increase in traditional marriages in recent decades.

Other common features of families in these countries are associated with their composition, values, and social roles. Extended family members tend to play a more central role in rural families, while relationships in nuclear families are emphasized more often in urban areas, especially among the middle class.[6] Childbearing is celebrated and very highly valued, which explains why Liberia and Sierra Leone have some of the world's highest fertility rates. Families in these countries are also patriarchal, with wives playing complementary roles to support their husbands. Although many wives participate in income-generating activities, husbands are usually the main breadwinners, especially among the poor, for whom sustenance is directly linked to their use of physical labor.

As in other contexts, deaths in African families affect not only the families' structure and composition but also their ability to perform these social roles. Consequently, deaths observed in families during periods of crisis, as well as the changes they engender, are among the most visible consequences of epidemics to the social structure of affected communities. These deaths contribute to changes in how families perform their traditional roles of fostering social cohesion, economic production, and cultural continuity. Moreover, they require families to help lessen the effects of crises on their members, which is why families bear much of the burden associated with recent civil conflicts and other humanitarian disasters in West Africa.

These impacts took on a new level of importance after the start of the Ebola epidemic, because families were the social institutions at the center of the response to the crisis. Part of this situation arose because of the fact that Ebola is a caregiver's disease.[7] At the outset of the crisis, this designation was used to highlight the significant risks of infection faced by health care professionals as they provided medical care for those infected. However, it soon became clear that families were the first providers of such care, especially in places with limited access to vehicles to take the sick to hospitals and places with high health care costs.[8] This position of families as the primary places of care made them vulnerable to high levels of viral transmission among their members. Subsequent death to family caregivers and their kin significantly reduced family sizes. Nevertheless, the full impact of Ebola deaths on families remains unknown because of the difficulties involved in accounting for the number of families that were completely eliminated by the disease.

Families affected by Ebola were further vulnerable to the tragic consequences of the disease because of the diversity of family relationships found within households. In Liberia and Sierra Leone, families usually live in households that include more than just parents and their children. Most households are multigenerational and include children (and/or their cousins), parents (and/or aunts and uncles), and grandparents. Because multigenerational households have larger numbers of residents, all it took for them to experience a mass mortality event was a single case of Ebola infection. Thereafter, a cascading series of virus transmissions produced complex patterns of mortality that involved the deaths of nuclear and extended family members living in the same household.

At the same time, families are among the first places where recovery from epidemics begins. After survivors returned home from ETUs, the primary sources of support they received as they started the process of rebuilding their lives were derived from family relationships. The amount of support they could receive depended on the number of family members who were still alive. This meant that the greatest obstacles to recovery were faced by survivors who lost all or most of their families. The rebuilding process within families, however, differed from those in other social institutions, such as schools, in several important ways. In comparison to these institutions, families started rebuilding earlier, with little or no support from international aid agencies, and were driven more by altruistic concerns. Overall, these differences underscore the unique strengths and vulnerabilities faced by families as they adjusted to the realities of life in a post-epidemic world.

Ebola and Its Consequences for Family Life

A good place to begin the examination of the families most affected by the 2014 epidemic is to articulate how they differ in composition, character, and dynamics compared to how they looked before the start of the crisis. The new household structures in which family life occurs for many survivors are a reflection of the high mortality consequences of the epidemic. Many of these consequences have been documented in studies conducted in Guinea, Liberia, and Sierra Leone that examine selected aspects of family life among Ebola survivors.[9] To provide a more systematic review of these issues, however, the review that follows draws information from two sources: an in-depth survey of the family life of Ebola survivors in Sierra Leone and a general survey of the lives of Ebola survivors in both Liberia and Sierra Leone.

Not surprisingly, the most extensive transformations in the family lives of survivors were found among those who had many Ebola deaths in their families. One representation of this was found in the case of Halima, the sole survivor among multiple individuals infected in her family in Sierra Leone. Absent in her decision to start describing these transformations by stating that she "lost too many people" was the fact that she was 1 of 24 people who were infected in her immediate and extended families. All of them lived in separate households in the same compound at the start of the epidemic. However, tragedy struck after Halima's husband became ill and started having symptoms such as frequent diarrhea and vomiting of blood. After family members stepped in to care for him, the disease spread to other residents of the compound. As a result, 23 of the 24 infected people died of Ebola, including Halima's husband, cousins, nieces, nephews, and some of her children.

Now living in different household circumstances, Halima describes who she considers to be the members of her family: "My aunt, who I live with, and her children. They are the ones assisting me now." She explained that she did not have anywhere to go after she recovered, because she lost so many members of her family. Her aunt offered to assist, and she allowed her to live with her family. However, the new arrangement was not ideal because of other related hardships. As a result, although she appreciated the hospitality of her aunt, she still faced constraints because her aunt was poor. Moreover, the household poverty she now experienced was in stark contrast to the more favorable economic circumstances in her former family. As she thought about these things she said, "I miss my husband because he was the one doing everything for me."

Survivors from small pre-epidemic families experienced similar familial transformations. Although the relative numbers of deaths in these families were fewer, they still had notable consequences. Jenneh, who now lived in a middle-class suburb of Freetown, was part of one such family at the start of the epidemic that consisted of five other individuals—her husband, their three children, and her cousin. She was the first in the group to contract the disease. During her stay in an ETU, she believed she was the only one in her family who had contracted the disease until she received a message saying that her husband had developed severe complications from Ebola. He died shortly thereafter, and his death was followed by that of her cousin.

Now raising the couple's three children on her own, Jenneh said she misses the emotional support of her husband the most, because she did not have to face their family challenges alone. Jenneh described the impacts of these deaths by saying:

> The death of my husband makes me lonely. Just imagine, I was still experiencing the trauma of Ebola when I heard the news; it caused more harm to me than good. Just imagine, you had a husband and he left you with the kids. I had three kids with him, and he is not here. It was hard for me to take care of the children. When he was alive, even when there was nothing in the house, because he had care and concern, I never had the feeling that we lacked anything. He used to do all he could to make sure that he takes care of the home, the children, and everything in the house. I lost all of this. I lost his care and concern.

Another part of her transition involved finding people who could step into roles previously played by her extended family members. Unlike Halima, who moved in with her aunt, Jenneh and her children were receiving help from others who can best be described as fictive kin. These fictive relationships are formed between individuals who regard each other as relatives although they are not related by blood or by marriage.[10] Accordingly, she clarified that her family included people who do more for her than a real family would normally do. For example, a woman she now calls her sister cries with her when she cries, provides food when she is hungry, and takes her to the hospital when she is ill.

As Ebola widows, Halima and Jenneh had one other common characteristic that defined their lives after the epidemic. They faced economic hardships they did not experience while their husbands were alive. Life after the death of a spouse can be particularly more daunting for women than for men in Africa due to gender disparities in economic attainment and cultural norms governing rights of inheritance. These norms make it difficult for widows to inherit their husband's resources. As a result, most of them experience declines in their economic status after the deaths of their spouses. Such declines are particularly notable in countries such as Sierra Leone. One study showed that among African widows, those in Sierra Leone were the least likely to receive a transfer of assets following the death of their husbands.[11] Part of this was because, in many cases, customary rights of inheritance give preferences to the parents and siblings of deceased husbands over surviving wives and children. Such practices only served to add to the challenges faced by Ebola widows as they tried to adjust to their new familial circumstances.

To provide a sense of how these rights are understood, Pat, a widow who lived on the outskirts of Freetown, described what happened after the death of her husband. Before he died of Ebola, they lived in a house he owned, along with their two children and her mother, aunt, and niece. All seven of them were subsequently infected with Ebola, but Pat was the only one who survived. Shortly after she returned home from an ETU, her husband's relatives asked her to move out of the house. The explanation they provided was annoyingly simple: Her husband was dead, so his house now belonged to them. They did not have any legal documents to support their claim, nor did Pat. Furthermore, she was still physically weak as she recovered from Ebola and did not want to endure the costly process of taking legal action against them. Without contesting their claim but with an understanding of how inheritance worked, she gave up the home and went to live with her uncle.

Such experiences underscore the gendered nature of the consequences of spousal death among Ebola survivors. Indeed, unlike their female counterparts, the economic circumstances of male survivors are rarely determined by the resources left behind by their deceased spouses. When men spoke about the consequences of the deaths of their spouses, they generally focused on a different set of issues than those captured in the narratives of women. When men spoke about life without their wives, they often highlighted the emotional consequences of these deaths, such as depression, confusion, and challenges raising their children. By contrast, women often focused on the economic consequences of the deaths of their husbands, such as the lack of resources to care for their children, in addition to the emotional toll of losing their husbands. These economic burdens were more significant among widows who lived in very poor communities. Among these women, spousal deaths were associated with taking on new economic responsibilities while also living in poverty.

For example, consider what happened to Musu, a woman in Monrovia, Liberia, who did not finish high school and is now a widow. Her original family of eight was devastated by the loss of the critical multigenerational relationships that existed in her household before it was struck by Ebola. The first person to be infected was her older daughter, a nurse who contracted the disease while treating a patient she did not know was already infected. After she became sick, seven other members of her family, including her five sons and her husband, also became infected. Of the original eight members of the family, Musu and one of her sons were the only survivors. In the absence of the support she would have received from her husband, she now faced notable economic constraints as she struggled with her new circumstances. She described them as follows:

> Of my five sons, only one is alive, but I can't pay his tuition. He is in the 10th grade and there is no one here to help besides God. No boyfriend. No father. I am the father, the mother, the uncle, and the brother. At the place we are renting, we can't even get food to eat every day. I worry about my son's education, but he is the only one living now.

When other Liberian widows discussed the impacts of their husbands' deaths, they also focused on similar social consequences. Spousal deaths left them without their usual sources of economic support, which was made much worse when their brothers-in-law also died of Ebola, because this eliminated an alternative source of support. Furthermore, when they transitioned to becoming the sole breadwinner, some widows in Liberia became responsible not only for their surviving children but also for orphans they fostered as a result of Ebola deaths among their relatives.

Changes in Relationships with Extended Family Members

While having surviving relatives can potentially help bereaved survivors in the process of rebuilding their lives, this assistance was not always forthcoming. In fact, the relationships survivors had with their extended families were complicated. Traditionally, these families provide social and economic support to members of their kin groups to help them rebound from tragedy. However, the social consequences of the epidemic were so far reaching that only a few survivors were able to leverage these relationships to improve their circumstances.

There were several reasons for this. First, as mentioned earlier, the clustering of Ebola deaths in multigenerational households eliminated arguably the closest candidates who could have played these traditional roles. Second, many of the remaining relatives were themselves Ebola survivors struggling to get back on their feet. Third, regardless of their prior Ebola status, many extended family members lived in the same state of poverty that continues to be widespread in the affected West African countries.

These resource limitations had particularly adverse consequences for families in poor communities. At the Susan's Bay slum, which hosts one of the poorest communities in Freetown, one survivor described the ironic way in which poverty shaped her relationship with the only extended family member on whom she could rely. She was one of five members of her immediate family who were infected with Ebola and one of only two people who survived. While she now struggles to make ends meet, her relationship with her extended family members is generally poor. The exception to this was her relationship was her aunt, who turned out to be more disadvantaged than she was. As she put it:

> The exception to this is my mother's older sister, but she also is poor. Her family is poor. In fact, we are the ones who sometimes help her with small cash donations. When we receive money given to us as Ebola survivors, we usually give her some of it because my mother was the person helping her when she was alive even though my aunt was the older one. My aunt is poor; that's why we don't depend on her.

When poverty was not a factor that limited the support survivors received from their relatives, these survivors still had to confront their relatives' lingering fears about continued Ebola infection. These fears weakened these relationships and did so to such an extent that some survivors chose to fend for themselves instead. A more important consequence of these fears was their negative impacts on social interactions between survivors and their relatives at large family events. The most frequent manifestations of these problems came in the form of declines in the number of invitations survivors received to social events such as marriages and child-naming ceremonies. In the worst of circumstances, family members no longer extended these invitations at all. When comparing her inclusion in these events before and after she contracted Ebola, one survivor said, "Before I had this sickness, we would be invited to weddings and naming ceremonies. We would go and have a good time. Since I had Ebola, [my relatives] no longer tell me. They do not come near me." In other cases, family members invited them to these events but did not welcome them. When they attended, many survivors could not help but notice the negative ways in which they were treated. As another survivor observed, "If I visit when a child is born, they act like they are afraid. They don't talk to me nicely."

Ebola, Broken Marriages, and Spousal Abandonment

Fears about the infectiousness of survivors were felt much closer to home, where they led to disruptions in marriages and romantic relationships. For the most part, these disruptions were observed among Ebola-discordant couples—that is, couples in which one individual contracted the disease and the other did not. For infected individuals, discordance meant that returning home from ETUs was no guarantee of a happy reunion with their waiting spouses. Instead, it frequently led to the abandonment of marriages, mostly by husbands who left their Ebola-surviving wives. Although their wives had recovered from their infections, the departing husbands assumed they were still infectious and were able to transmit the disease to others. What made this worse was the fact that these departures seemed to be permanent. In fact, no survivor who participated in the study reported that a partner who previously abandoned them had subsequently returned. Because these relationships were permanently broken, abandoned spouses continued to live with experiences of grief, a loss of status, and in socioeconomic circumstances quite similar to those observed among widows.

As Fola, a survivor who faced these realities, described in her account of being abandoned after she returned home from an ETU, the experience can be extremely stressful. Before being discharged, she celebrated her recovery with nurses and other health care workers, only to have her joyous mood tempered by her husband's response when she got home. Recalling what happened, she said, "After I returned home, he abandoned me. He was afraid of me, so he ran away and left me with the children." At the time of his departure, Fola had close relatives who were still infected with Ebola and admitted to a hospital. Therefore, she went through the arduous process of juggling her concerns about whether they would survive, her own apprehensions about her fragile health, and the shattered marriage caused by her husband's decision. Her explanation of what happened next underlined the vulnerabilities survivors faced as they dealt with these issues. As she stated, "What my husband did made me so frustrated that I got sick again. I had fevers. I took Panadol until I got better. I had a lot on my mind, so I became depressed. I had to go to the MSF clinic for treatment. The MSF people counseled me until I returned to normal."

Fola's mental health later improved, but her relationship with her husband did not. Additionally, she began to experience the economic consequences of his departure almost immediately after he left. In the following weeks, things got so bad that the only food she had was what was offered to her by her younger sister. She now lived as a single mother in the town of Waterloo, where she continues to face hardships she associates with her husband's abandonment. For example, she has not been able to find an alternative source of capital to replace what he used to provide for her to conduct her business. Her limited years of schooling have compounded the problem. Because she left school in the fourth grade, she has found it difficult to secure a stable source of income to support herself and her children.

However, Fola's experience is not unique. Nearby is another survivor named Binta, who was abandoned by her spouse in circumstances slightly different from Fola's. In Binta's case, the Ebola-related problems in her marriage started before she became infected, after she learned that her mother was ill. Upon receiving the news, she informed her husband that she planned to visit her mother's residence to take care of her. She did not know at the time that her mother had already contracted Ebola, and neither did her husband. She had heard public health messages asking the public not to care for sick people at home but to take them to the hospital instead. However, she ignored them so she could care for her mother personally. When her husband learned that his mother-in-law was actually infected with Ebola, he became so upset that he decided to end the marriage. Shortly thereafter, Binta was infected with the disease, but she recovered.

After her husband's departure, Binta moved to her current community, where she lives alone in a rundown house. She lost the occasional economic support she received from her parents after they both died of Ebola. With no bed to sleep on as she did when she was married, she now slept on a cold floor. Reflecting on how her living circumstances have changed since the epidemic, she said, "When my [parents] were still alive, I used to get what I want, but now I have nothing. I am sleeping on the floor. I have nothing. I survive by things people give to me out of sympathy. I don't have a child. I have lost my relatives. I don't have anyone. I don't have a partner, nor do I have relatives who are helping me."

Rebuilding Romantic Relationships

One potential option for rebuilding family life after widowhood or separation is to start by forming new romantic relationships. Many survivors had a desire to start such relationships, and their reasons for this were diverse. Some framed these desires in instrumental terms focusing on the advantages of having someone to share the economic burden of raising a family and help around the house. Others mainly wanted companionship and needed to take a step toward returning to normal. This desire to start romantic relationships was found not only among survivors who were previously married but also among younger survivors who were thinking about the possibility of starting their first families.

Success in forming these relationships, however, is very rare. A few survivors who were involved in romantic relationships before they became infected were fortunate to have their partners remain by their side as they recovered. More common, however, was single survivors facing heartbreaking disappointments as they interacted with potential partners. Possible partners were still attracted but reacted negatively after they learned about the survivors' medical history.

Jenneh, who lost her husband to Ebola, shared her encounters with these experiences after she started dating again. Seven months after she returned home from the hospital, she met someone she liked a lot. As they got to know each other, during a visit to her home, the person casually asked her if she knew anyone who was an Ebola survivor. It was the first time the issue had come up, so she responded honestly and disclosed that she was a survivor. To her shock, "He left my house and never returned. He said he did not want to have Ebola and that he did not want to die at an early age."

Stella, a 24-year-old survivor who had never married, agreed that it was difficult to have romantic relationships as an Ebola survivor. Her first experience with this occurred after she was discharged from the hospital and involved a boyfriend she referred to as a "brother in church," who initially had planned to propose marriage. However, after she returned home in January 2015, he phoned her to end the relationship. The boyfriend was forthcoming about his reason: He was concerned about her previous Ebola infection. Stella said this experience left her feeling stressed.

Other accounts of young women attempting to date after Ebola pointed to a pattern of cognitive dissonance among the potential boyfriends they encountered. On the one hand, these men did not desire stable relationships with female survivors because of their previous experience with the disease. On the other hand, they had no problem expressing their interest in sleeping with survivors to satisfy their sexual needs. One Ebola widow who began dating after the death of her husband was quick to recognize the disconnection between the short-term actions and the long-term intentions of these men. She explained the following:

> Some of them come and ask you to be their girlfriend, but when they ask around about me, people tell them that I am an Ebola survivor. They just come and have sex with you and leave you. So, I just stopped doing that. I'll just wait for a good man. If I don't find one, I would pray to God for something good in my life. Men are afraid of us because they say we have been sick with Ebola.

Other young survivors who had never been married encountered similar situations. For example, a 24-year-old woman who lost 5 members of her family said men wanted to sleep with her but were uninterested in having a long-term relationship. She found this disconcerting, saying she was not as hopeful as her peers who had decided to wait for a good man. She was so negatively affected by these behaviors that she decided to stop dating, saying, "I don't want that. That's why I don't have time for men." However, she continued, "My life is not great. I sometimes pretend, but I am not happy," expressing sadness at the realization of her somewhat hopeless situation.

Notwithstanding the fact that the fear of Ebola was an impediment to dating, it was not the only factor that negatively affected the likelihood of successfully entering romantic relationships. Widows with children found it very difficult to find partners who were willing to consider the prospect of dealing with future stepchildren. Through tears, one of them described how this had affected her ability to have boyfriends. She was still raising the five children she had with her deceased husband. When she met potential suitors, some of them expressed interest in a relationship, until they learn about her children. For other widows, the main impediment was the fact that they were still mourning their spouses. They spoke of how difficult it was to find someone who had the same characteristics as their spouse and who meant as much to them. Finally, a few others said they were not at the point of considering romantic relationships, and much of their hesitation was due to the fear of rejection by potential partners.

Parental Deaths and Their Consequences for Children

Changes in the family circumstances of adults provide just one perspective on the social consequences of the epidemic. Another perspective is provided by examining how these consequences affected the familial circumstances of the surviving children. One such child is Fatu, a young lady who said she was infected with Ebola as a teenager. What remains of her household in Freetown is now quite different from what it was before the epidemic. Back then, her household was like many in the city—a dynamic collection of immediate and extended family members that included a set of grandparents, her siblings, a cousin, and her parents. All of this changed after her cousin became sick with a high fever and started vomiting frequently. They soon learned he had contracted Ebola from a friend, who, in turn, was infected by his girlfriend. Her father, a medical doctor, became sick after contracting the disease from a patient.

As Fatu now admits, after her family found out that her cousin was infected, they refused to take him to the hospital but chose to provide care for him at home instead. As a result, the disease spread within their household, with the first person-to-person transmission occurring after her brother interacted with her cousin. After the death of her cousin, members of the family knew they were in trouble because so many of them had come into contact with him. Within 21 days, all 9 members of the household began showing symptoms of Ebola. Of this number, only Fatu and her younger sibling survived.

Since then, Fatu has become one of the many Ebola orphans who lost their parents during the epidemic, and her orphanhood has created two major changes in her social status. First, she is now the head of a new household consisting of five younger Ebola orphans, including her sibling and her cousins. Second, she is no longer the child of wealthy middle-class parents who were known in their community for their generosity. With no other source of support as she faced her new responsibilities, she left school to care for the young children, thereby placing their welfare above her own.

Estimates suggest that approximately 16,000 children were orphaned in the 2014 West African Ebola outbreak.[12] Some of these children have experienced far worse changes in the circumstances of their families compared to Fatu. The reasons for this should now be familiar: They are not just children who tragically lost their parents. Like many Ebola survivors, they experienced complex mortality losses within their families. Thus, the death of their parents was followed by that of other relatives and even older siblings who could have provided care for them in the absence of their parents. Furthermore, like other survivors, when they had surviving relatives, these relatives were usually too poor to provide them with any kind of assistance. These are some of the reasons why orphans are considered to be the most vulnerable victims of the Ebola epidemic.[13]

It is important to put the scale of orphanhood during the epidemic in its proper perspective. The estimated number of Ebola orphans represents only a small proportion of the overall number of orphans in the countries most affected by the epidemic because of their respective histories of civil conflict and the HIV epidemic.[14] Because extended family networks absorbed much of the orphan burden before the Ebola crisis, some have suggested that these networks should play a major role in dealing with the epidemic's aftermath. Although this expectation is reasonable, it understates the unique social consequences of Ebola infections. In multigenerational households, for example, a single exposure to Ebola is likely to lead to more deaths than a single exposure to HIV/AIDS. Moreover, compared to children orphaned by HIV/AIDS or by conflict, Ebola orphans are arguably more likely to face higher levels of stigma, which can have adverse implications for their integration into society.

These factors have combined to negatively affect the lives of Ebola orphans and forced many of them to the margins of society. A few of them have been relatively fortunate to be institutionalized in the many orphanages that sprung up in the affected countries at the end of the epidemic. However, these orphanages lack the capacity to address the needs of all orphans. For example, one estimate indicates that there are only 48 residential institutions in Sierra Leone to care for a total of 1,100 vulnerable children, including orphans.[15] However, the country is believed to have more than 300,000 orphans.[16] Similarly, Liberia is believed to have 114 orphanages, but estimates indicate that close to 80% of children living in them have one living parent.[17] Like many other orphans, therefore, children orphaned by Ebola generally live in non-institutionalized contexts, and their marginalization is particularly evident among those who are now homeless.

Few Ebola orphans represented these experiences as much as Fatima and her friend Memuna. Both are illiterate and live on the streets near a busy transportation terminal in Freetown. When Fatima was told at the ETU that she had fully recovered from the disease, her joy was tempered by the realization of the significant challenges that lay ahead because she had lost both her parents. She initially went to her relatives for help, and they agreed to let her live with them. However, their fear of Fatima became obvious when she was asked to move into a room no one dared to pass by, located at the back of the house. When she got tired of how she was ostracized, she left the house to start life on the streets of Freetown. As she described what happened in the following remarks, it became clear that her life took a turn for the worse after she became homeless:

> After I started living on the streets, I gave birth to two children. The father of the children and I are now separated. He does not know what's going on with them. The place where we sleep is dry. We sleep on cardboards here. Now, I am selling peanuts to live my life. My brothers do not want to know about me. The

babies' father sometimes come with 10, 20, or 50 thousand leones,[18] but it's better than nothing. However, I still pray to God because God helps makes things better, so that's how I survive.

The plight of her friend Memuna was similar to hers in the sense that they both lost their parents. Unlike Fatima, however, Memuna did not have the luxury of spending even a short time with her relatives after she was released from the ETU. In part, this was because she was diagnosed with Ebola when she was a teenager living in Kono, which is located 225 miles from Freetown, and was completely abandoned by her relatives after she became an orphan. Left with no other option than to live alone, she decided to move to Freetown, where she had a better chance of surviving, since Freetown is the capital city. She now lives on the streets.

According to Memuna, she does not keep in touch with her relatives. For now, her family consists of herself, her partner, who is also homeless, and a baby they just had together. Her account of the plight of her homeless family provides additional insight into the consequences of experiencing homelessness in Freetown:

> Up until this moment, I do not have a place to sleep. I usually sleep over there [a corner on the side of the street] near where my partner sleeps. That's where we spread cardboards at night and sleep. When it rains, the place where we sleep gets wet. I just sit there holding my child while crying, because if my mother was alive, this would not have happened. My mum would have helped take care of the child. Now, because of the low temperatures, my child sometimes has a cold. I also have my sleep interrupted a lot. By 4 a.m. . . . in the morning, the traders start arriving to start their day. When they do, we have to pack up the cardboards and get ready to leave. When this happens, my sleep is interrupted, and my child's sleep is interrupted.

Lacking support from her relatives back in Kono, Memuna has had to depend more on the relatives of her partner. Even though they were also poor, her relatives shared their meager resources with Memuna and made her feel that she is one of them. However, the relationship is far from ideal. For one, it does not replace the support she used to receive from her parents, whom she admits she still misses. Additionally, occasional conflicts with her in-laws only help to underscore the fragile nature of their relationship. When things get heated between them, she maintains, her in-laws deliberately say bad things about her deceased mother, which retraumatizes her and makes her cry when she remembers all the things she has been through.

It is not clear how Fanta and Memuma's lack of formal schooling at the time they became orphans adds to their current predicament. What is clear is that any chance they may have had of starting school has been all but eliminated by the deaths of their parents. This conclusion is based on research revealing that orphan status is associated with poor enrollment outcomes in many parts of Africa.[19] Other orphans, such as Fatu, who is caring for younger orphans, were forced to drop out of school after losing their parents. However, in Fatu's case, she quickly transitioned into playing a parent-like role to the young children in her household and focusing her attention on their own schooling. She is now the person they turn to when they need something for school, so to meet these and other needs, she does odd jobs for families who have more resources. She summarized her new responsibilities by stating the obvious: "These are not things I am used to doing. I can't do anything for myself, because any small amount of money I have is used to buy things to cook."

A few Ebola orphans have nevertheless been able to continue with their education with the help of wealthy benefactors, some of whom were friends of their parents. Others have continued their education with remarkable displays of resilience in the face of tremendous odds. These cases were rare, and one such rarity was reflected in the experiences of a young man called Musa, from a family of 11 people struck with Ebola after his father became infected. He was 17 at the time and was the only one in the family who survived. These events occurred when he was in the final year of secondary school, but he was determined to graduate. His determination motivated him to undertake odd jobs and other responsibilities at a local market to pay for his education, the costs of which were previously covered by his mother.

Musa was able to successfully complete secondary school, and then he decided to take on the greater challenge of attending college. Things became even more difficult, and this was one of the first times he realized that the disadvantage of having poor relatives extended beyond their lack of financial resources. Musa described how his lack of social connections torpedoed his effort to secure a government scholarship that pays the full tuition for college students. He applied for the scholarship but did not receive it; however, as was common in the flawed government bureaucracy in the country, a few students he knew received the grant even though they had not applied.[20] Musa, therefore, saw the difference between his failure and their successes from one perspective. Unlike those who succeeded, he did not have social connections with adults who could have advocated for him. In fact, such advocacy efforts would not have been needed if his mother had been alive. Still undeterred by these events, he was able to successfully gain admission to college. However, he now had an outstanding tuition bill he had no way of paying.

Although the preceding analysis drew on a survey of survivor families in Sierra Leone, the evidence collected from Liberia indicated that Liberian children orphaned by Ebola had similar familial experiences. Like their counterparts in Sierra Leone, they were disadvantaged by the loss of support from their parents as well as from their relatives who died from the disease. As a result, they faced crucial economic constraints that led many to drop out of school. The accounts of these orphans further revealed the extensive emotional toll of orphanhood, particularly the feelings of loneliness and trauma triggered by memories of their parents. As one male who was orphaned indicated, the world he now lived in looked strange because he no longer had anyone to help him. This change in their outlook on life was one of the many commonalities in the experiences of orphans in both countries.

Family Transitions and Disrupted Futures

All the evidence reviewed thus far points to one conclusion about how the families of Ebola survivors have fared since the epidemic ended. Overall, the cumulative effects of Ebola mortality on these families have been very negative. What does this mean in practical terms, and what are the instrumental pathways through which these impacts have shaped the life chances of survivors? A useful strategy employed by survivors to address these issues was to reflect on how they believed their lives would have been different had they not lost their loved ones to Ebola. As they articulated these differences, it became evident that the most important consequence of these deaths was their negative impact on survivors' socioeconomic mobility. This consequence was experienced in two ways.

The first was through the loss of the mobility-promoting resources that their families enjoyed before the epidemic. These losses did not necessarily lead to socioeconomic declines but simply prevented families from advancing. Therefore, survivors with these experiences were able to maintain a semblance of their former lifestyles but struggled with occasional hardships as they attempted to move on with their lives. This perspective was best articulated by a widow who said her husband did everything for her while he was alive. As she compared how things were before the epidemic with her current circumstances, she described how she was "making progress when [her] family members were alive," but then "everything broke down. Nothing [was] going forward." Now, she said, her main reasons for hope are the prayers she says, asking God to assist her.

The second way in which socioeconomic mobility was affected is related to the first. It started with the inability to make progress and concluded in a complete reversal of survivors' fortunes. When they talked about these reversals, survivors further placed them in context by identifying the possible goals that could have been achieved if no one had died in their families. For example, Memuna, who is now homeless, stated that had her parents lived, she would have had the opportunity to attend school, graduate from college, and look for work. This did not sound realistic seven years after the epidemic, since she had never been to school in that time. She could not help but observe how much worse her life had become after the deaths of her parents. As she put it, "My life in the past compared to now is different. Look at my condition. I am now sleeping on the streets."

Perceived reversals in life circumstances were further acknowledged by survivors who had been abandoned by their husbands. Unjust rules about the distribution of resources after divorce or separation in traditional marriages had made it difficult for them to continue their lives on solid footing. The lack of alternative sources of assistance due to the deaths of other close family members made it impossible to maintain their former lifestyles. Faced with this combination of challenges, Binta confidently concluded that her life was now worse because of the epidemic. She believed that, at the very least, she would have become "somebody in the community" if her parents were alive, even without her husband's help. Although she now slept on the floor of a house and paid rent she could barely afford, her parents would have helped her move to a better neighborhood where she would have enjoyed more opportunities. Moreover, they would have provided her with the resources she needed to pay the rent for her dilapidated house. Neither of these options was available, and as a result, her living conditions were now much worse than they were before the epidemic.

Other survivors orphaned by Ebola used the progress made by their non-orphaned friends as a yardstick to envision the life they, too, could have had. One of them talked about how sad she felt after learning that her childhood friend's dad had paid for her to travel to the Middle East to purchase goods to start a business. It was a life-changing opportunity she insisted her mother would have provided for her. She was confident that "instead of letting me sit idly by, [her mother] would have paid for me to travel to do business in places like Oman and Turkey." She put this confidence in perspective by describing the closeness of their relationship. Her mother was the one who paid her school fees and was the person she described as the biggest influence in her life. The relationship between them was so close that, when her mother contracted Ebola, she became her main caregiver. After her parents' death, she was kicked out of their family home, left school, and was now homeless.

Although many Ebola orphans lost both parents, most of them talked about their mothers when discussing the monumental changes that had occurred in their life circumstances. This is partly due to the economic role played by mothers, who in some cases covered the cost of school fees. However, the majority of the reasons orphans gave for missing their mothers were non-economic. For example, the loss of their mothers was associated with the absence of warm meals, happiness at home, and other factors one survivor referred to as "mom stuff." By "mom stuff," she was referring to the new responsibility she now had to raise her younger sister, who was the only other person in her family of seven who survived after they were all infected with Ebola. Without her mother to do the "mom stuff," she said, she was "finding it difficult to do certain things; even training up my younger sister is difficult." In fact, she was now playing the roles of both mother and sister to her younger sibling, which was something she struggled with. It was not part of the future she had imagined for herself while her mother was still alive.

Families and the Social Dimensions of Recovery

Prior exposure to Ebola infections within families has had far-reaching implications for the lives of survivors in the years following the epidemic. The families they now have are generally configured differently than the families they had in the past. At the same time, their new families have struggled to perform many of their traditional functions while facing significant challenges as they attempt to recover from the crisis. Deaths within households led to the loss of breadwinners and sources of emotional support. When such deaths occurred in multigenerational households, they eliminated alternative sources of support survivors could have utilized to help them rebound from the crisis. Most of these structural and social changes that occurred in the families of survivors are irreversible. What's more, they have exposed survivors to new sources of adversity that have significant social implications.

The consequences of these adversities have been diverse. They include the loss of status that accompanies the collapse of marriages and the loss of significant others. Widows have experienced rejection from their in-laws, while single women are no longer considered desirable for long-term romantic relationships. The loss of social status has also led to the exclusion of survivors from familial events such as marriages and has made it difficult for them to develop meaningful relationships with their surviving relatives.

Changes in the dynamics of families have further increased the social vulnerability of survivors. The group most affected by these vulnerabilities are orphans, many of whom have joined the ranks of marginalized people enduring homelessness. Equally important patterns of vulnerability in the families of survivors helped to push them into worse economic circumstances. The resources available within their new families have been more limited compared to those they had before the epidemic. Consequently, families that were formerly self-sufficient have been pushed into poverty, while those that were poor have been made poorer still. Any economic vulnerability in their families before the epidemic has been worsened; widows have trouble providing for their children, and orphans have had to drop out of school.

It should not be difficult to see how the evidence reviewed thus far underscores the need for systematic social responses to the consequences of the epidemic. If families are to achieve meaningful success in the Ebola recovery efforts they started well before other institutions, such responses are needed. Without them, however, families have found their own ways of being resilient. They have leaned on the resources of fictive kin, performed parental roles while caring for their siblings, and steered away from strained relationships with relatives. In other words, Ebola survivors have demonstrated agency in responding to the disruptive effects of the epidemic on their families Yet these responses have not been enough to address other long-term challenges they continue to experience.

4 The Health Consequences
of Prior Ebola Infection

Before Teta decided to get tested for Ebola, she spent a few days at home treating her suspected symptoms of the disease. She did not want to believe that she was already infected. However, her training as a health care worker suggested otherwise. As a result, when her symptoms failed to improve, she went to the John F. Kennedy (JFK) Hospital in Monrovia to finally get tested. The result confirmed what she feared. It was positive for Ebola. Consequently, she was admitted for three weeks at the hospital's ETU. At the end of this period, she was discharged and given an official certificate indicating that she was now Ebola-free. To a large extent, however, this freedom was fleeting. It simply marked the beginning of a new phase in her life that involved dealing with complications related to the sequelae (aftereffects) of the disease.

This new phase started after Teta returned home from the hospital. The first few days were rough because she continued feeling weak, while her health declined. At one point, Teta felt as sick as she did when initially admitted as an Ebola patient. After that, her health worsened so much that her friends began to stay away from her, thinking she still had the disease. The tipping point came when she eventually became blind. Concerned about the loss of her eyesight, her brother called the JFK Hospital intending to get her readmitted. During the call, he was informed that he did not need to bring her in because Teta was indeed Ebola-free and that her loss of eyesight was temporary. Consistent with this prediction, she began to see again in the following weeks. However, despite this improvement, Teta started to deal with new chronic conditions she did not have before. They included problems with her eyes that required her to use prescription glasses.

Additionally, she started having joint pains and severe headaches, all of which combined to negatively affect her quality of life.

Today, many Ebola survivors, like Teta, face health problems associated with their prior experience with the disease. The specific types of problems they encounter are diverse. They include chronic pains, mental health complications, and skin diseases, as well as other health concerns. The scale of these health complications is so extensive that it was believed to have contributed to an "emergency within the emergency."[1] While no one doubts that the public health emergency observed during the 2014 epidemic has ended, an ongoing emergency still exists, defined by the many health issues being experienced by survivors. Unlike the 2014 crisis, which attracted significant attention from health policymakers, attention to the latter has been limited. As a result, it has continued to transform the burden of disease of the countries that were affected by the epidemic.

These transformations represent a critical component of the social dimensions of the epidemic's aftermath. Comparing the response to these transformations to those observed during the 2014 epidemic provides one way of examining how medical responses differ from social responses. During the epidemic, the medical response to the crisis resulted in a massive infusion of resources in the form of the medical equipment, drugs, and health care personnel from abroad. Since then, the primary medical responses have focused on meso-level interventions, such as developing new vaccines and constructing effective disease surveillance systems. At the micro-level, however, the response to the needs of survivors has been limited. To make things worse, very little attention has been given to the social transformations that have resulted from the negative impact of the disease's sequelae on the incorporation of survivors into their communities.

Such transformations have been observed in the lives of many survivors recovering from infections in prior epidemics. While their exposure to disease provided them with some form of immunity to specific infections, their recovery is usually followed by a long-term process of dealing with the sequelae of the disease. For example, in his classic work on the historic Plague of Athens, Thucydides observed that many of its survivors eventually succumbed to blindness, gangrene infections, memory loss, and other diseases.[2]

However, the specific disease sequelae observed across epidemics vary.

Survivors of smallpox and polio epidemics have been found to have high rates of blindness and paralysis, while those of rubella epidemics tended to have high rates of deafness.[3] More recent evidence from the COVID-19 pandemic further shows the continued significance of these patterns. In particular, infection from the disease increases the risk of experiencing various complications now collectively known as Long COVID. People afflicted by Long COVID have high levels of suicidal behavior,[4] shortness of breath, and depression.[5]

Survivors of epidemics tend to adjust to life with new health complications in a process that is inherently social. It requires them to draw support from social networks that have often been depleted or no longer exist. The process shapes their social interactions through health problems that limit how they move, their access to resources, and their participation in social institutions. Further, new chronic conditions have other immediate social implications in the form of constraints to survivors' ability to perform their usual activities of daily living. Moreover, these conditions require them to develop new health-seeking behaviors to help them navigate their various challenges.

Understanding the social dimensions of the health problems confronted by Ebola survivors requires an examination of the various manifestations of the medical complications they now face as well as the social implications of living with these conditions. The connection between the two is crucial because it helps us assess how well survivors have been integrated into their communities. In addition, examining these connections is critical for assessing whether the social response to the consequences of the epidemic has been adequate. To conduct this assessment, it is important to answer a number of questions. For example, how have the health complications of Ebola survivors changed over time? In what ways have these conditions affected their participation in social life? How have social institutions responded to their diverse medical needs? Finally, what are the major patterns of health-seeking behavior used by survivors to address their ongoing health challenges?

Returning Home But Not in Full Health

One of the first things Ebola survivors realize after they return home from the hospital is that recovery takes time. Adjusting to this reality tends to be a two-phase process. The first involves dealing with the effects of the physical toll of the Ebola infection, which they experienced in the weeks before they were discharged. For example, losing bodily fluids from diarrhea and vomiting can lead to dramatic weight loss that leaves most survivors emaciated when they are discharged. The second is the start of a longer-term process of recovery that involves dealing with new chronic health conditions.

The first phase can leave community members confused; Most survivors continue to experience the symptoms they had when they were infected. In some cases, their physical appearance after returning home is not that different from what it was before they were taken to a hospital. As a result, it is easy for neighbors to harbor suspicions about whether survivors who have just been discharged have truly recovered from the disease. Such concerns are similar to that expressed by Teta's brother, who called the JFK Hospital to get her readmitted.

Bami, another survivor who was treated at the same hospital, faced similar concerns that spread within his community, especially when he became ill just after he returned home. At the time, his body was still reacting to some of the drugs he took while admitted. Viewing his illness as evidence of his continued infection with Ebola, his neighbors organized to take him to the hospital forcefully. Fortunately, a team of health workers visiting the community at the time prevented them from doing so.

Some survivors believe there is a direct connection between the illnesses they experienced immediately after returning home and the specific treatments they received at ETUs. One, for example, blamed a skin condition she had for several weeks on the medications Cotrim and Septrine, which she received at an ETU. Others mentioned that they went home with vision problems caused by the extensive use of chlorine to prevent the spread of Ebola within ETUs. Some support for this suspicion has been found in existing studies. Research suggests that the extensive use of chlorine to disinfect ETUs during the epidemic was positively associated with the risk of developing eye, respiratory, and skin-related conditions.[6]

As with Teta, most cases of blindness experienced by survivors after they returned home were temporary. Another survivor in Liberia, for example, maintained that he lost sight in his left eye after returning home, but only for two weeks. Apart from the possible effects of exposure to chlorine, temporary vision loss was also caused by the virus itself. In one case, for example, a survivor lost his vision a month after returning but regained his vision after the problem was treated with medication. He maintained that his doctor informed him that his temporary vision loss was caused by traces of the virus that were still in his eyes.

Other short-term ailments experienced by survivors following their discharge were associated with the pains they still had from therapies they received while they were ill. For example, according to one survivor, the short-term pain he experienced one week after returning home from the hospital resulted from what he referred to as a "big, big needle" injected into his body. Such physical pains were not always experienced in isolation but were symptoms that disappeared relatively quickly.

Among people hardest hit by the virus, recovery from these pains did not always occur quickly. One example of this was found in the experience of Alphia, whose pain symptoms started while she was admitted to the Eternal Love Winning Africa (ELWA) hospital in Monrovia, Liberia. Recalling what happened during this period, she explained that she was so weak after she was discharged that it was sometimes impossible for her to get down from her bed. The pains continued for several months after she was discharged. Describing what she went through during the process, she said, "I would lie down because I could not walk . . . I was helpless, even to get up from the bed, it was not easy for me. This happened on and off until the middle part of the year before I started feeling like I had recovered."

Returning home for other survivors was accompanied by the onset of new complications that marked the start of a more extended journey of dealing with various chronic ailments. One such transition was reported by Max, a construction worker in Monrovia's Montserrado County, who had what he thought was a temporary illness that had now become a chronic condition. Max returned home after being discharged from the ELWA Hospital, only to begin experiencing a frequent burning sensation he had never felt before. According to him:

The first side effect I experienced—and up to now it is still disturbing me—was a feeling of hotness under my feet. It felt like a severe burning, a burning that extends to as far as my back, coming towards my spine, and then moving directly to my chest, which makes it become very heavy. Up to now I still get the burning sensation on my thigh coming toward my neck. I have even decided to go for a check-up to know whether it is because I have a problem with my appendix. I haven't received the actual result. However, up to now, when I even stand for five minutes, I feel a severe burning pain.

Max's account captures only one way in which the transition to living with chronic health conditions occurred. Indeed, the onset of the second phase of recovery is far more complex than the onset of the first phase. In some cases, it starts immediately after survivors return home, but in others, in subsequent weeks. However, in all cases, this phase of recovery is observed over multiple years and continued to be experienced at the time of the interviews. Many of these chronic conditions also occurred as co-morbidities alongside other long-term medical complications of Ebola.

Furthermore, while it is tempting to examine these complications from a strictly medical perspective, it is essential to remember that they are being experienced by survivors with other socioeconomic disadvantages that shape their respective experiences. Each of these conditions is important in its own right and affects the survivors' recovery in different ways. Nevertheless, a general sense of their dynamics can be developed by focusing on some of those most frequently experienced by survivors since the end of the epidemic.

Mental Health and Neurological Complications

As Seray talked about the day she was released from an ETU in Freetown, you could tell she was happy that her ordeal was over. She had contracted Ebola from her husband, who later died of the disease. Since his death, she has lived the life of a widow attempting to rebound from her adversity. Like other survivors, she experienced chronic pains in the days following her return home from the ETU. However, the issue that was of utmost concern to her relatives was the state of her mental health. It was a concern driven by Seray's new tendency to talk to herself, because this was not something they had observed before.

Along with this new behavior, her eyes were occasionally red, possibly from eye complications related to her prior infection. As a result of these changes, residents in her community began to refer to her as a madwoman. Labeling her as such subjected her to scorn and laughter, the usual community reactions to people considered insane. On some occasions, the harassment declined with the intervention of community leaders. On other occasions, she has defended herself by explaining to those making fun of her that her mental health problems started while she was mourning the death of her husband.

These experiences capture only some of the new mental health challenges Ebola survivors face on their journey to recovery. Various estimates have been given to capture the prevalence of these challenges. However, they tend to focus on specific mental health issues. For example, one estimate indicates that about 20% of all Ebola survivors in Liberia and Sierra Leone and 13% of those in Guinea meet the criteria for a diagnosis of depression.[7] Overall, the mental problems found among survivors are serious, and some scholars suggest the situation has reached the threshold for being considered a crisis.[8]

Mental health issues are, however, among the most complicated chronic medical conditions found among Ebola survivors, for several reasons. The first is that they manifest in diverse patterns, including symptoms of depression, anxiety, and the experience of memory loss. Another is that they stem from both the direct and indirect consequences of Ebola infection. Infection by the virus has been directly linked to neurological complications, which could affect mental health.[9] These neurological complications have increased survivors' risk of experiencing seizures, headaches, memory loss, and cranial abnormalities.[10] Other mental health challenges experienced by survivors are part of the indirect consequences of epidemics, such as the traumas associated with the loss of loved ones.

Like other chronic conditions experienced by survivors, these mental health complications rarely occur in isolation. As observed in the case of Seray, they can be experienced by individuals with chronic pains, vision problems, and social disadvantages such as widowhood. Regardless of how mental health conditions are experienced, however, their overall effect is the same. They create new health burdens that did not exist before the epidemic and limit survivors' ability to resume their normal activities.

These limitations are extensively captured in the accounts of survivors, even in instances when they lack the terminology needed to describe their problems as neurological or mental health conditions.[11] One Sierra Leonean survivor, for example, casually described how he started having spells of dizziness after he was discharged. Since then, his health complications have escalated to the point where he now experiences excruciating headaches. To begin his account of his experiences, he described some of his specific symptoms as well as how they affected his well-being: "[They] bother me a lot. When the sun is up, I feel pain in the middle of my head like it is boiling. When it hurts, blood runs down my nose . . . I had never experienced any of this before."

More generally, however, memory loss was the most common mental health problem. It was a symptom more frequently experienced by survivors who reported persistent headaches, although it is unclear whether there is a connection between the two. Miatta, an Ebola survivor in Liberia, provided a fascinating account of these symptoms and directly traced their origins to the day she was discharged. She was a cosmetic trader in Monrovia before she was infected and spent about three weeks at an ETU before she recovered.

The first time she experienced memory loss was while preparing to return home after being discharged. Taking us back to the day she was discharged, she described the experience as follows: "I was happy when I was coming home. I was happy, but I couldn't remember where I lived although I could remember the name of the area. I told the people, 'I can't remember the place, but I know the name of the area,' so they asked me where, [and I told them], and after that they put me in the car." The problem persisted in subsequent years, during which she experienced more frequent headaches and episodes of memory loss. Thus, when specifically asked whether she continues to experience any symptoms of illness or side effects of treatment, her response was: "Yes, the headaches, and now as I am speaking to you, my head is still hurting. Since the day I recovered, I have suffered from headaches and forgetfulness. I forget too much."

Mental health issues associated with the traumatic experiences of survivors resulted in other significant behavioral changes. The primary group of people with such experiences were orphans, widows, and others who lost loved ones to Ebola. Among this group, accounts of mental health problems frequently described experiences with bouts of depression, which were triggered by memories of the deceased, and feelings of loneliness.

Other traumas were related to survivors' prior experiences as patients at ETUs that were now associated with new forms of anxiety. One survivor in Sierra Leone maintained that she had symptoms of anxiety driven by memories of being taken to the ETU in an ambulance. As a result of this, the sound of ambulance sirens now made her sick. It was a reaction that started shortly after she returned home, and although she had learned to deal with the worst of these symptoms, the problem persisted. Consequently, she said,

> Any time I hear an ambulance, I feel sick and become nervous. I need someone to calm me down until it passes by. It took a while before my reaction to it subsided. In the past, when I hear an ambulance, I would start shaking and breathing heavily. Because I think of the day the ambulance came to pick me up when I had Ebola. Since that time, I always feel stressed when I hear an ambulance.

Collectively, the mental health complications of survivors have had negative implications for their ability to perform their usual functions. The most prevalent of these were related to the problem of memory loss, headaches, and occasional spells of dizziness. Memory loss contributed to minor inconveniences such as "searching for something around the house while holding it in your hand" and temporarily forgetting the names of parents. Some of the more severe implications included the limits placed by memory loss on survivors' ability to participate in school or work-related activities. For one eleventh-grade student, the problem created new obstacles for him after returning to school because class lessons that should have been easy to understand were now more difficult. New problems with his eyesight made this worse and also made it hard for him to read.

Another student provided a more telling account of the effects of her mental health and related symptoms. She reported that her frequent headaches and spells of dizziness were sometimes so severe that she periodically thought of skipping school. However, she was concerned that her dad would be disappointed if she did. Therefore, she explained, "Even if I am dizzy or sick, I still go to school. I don't want him to think I am staying home because I have done something wrong at school." She managed her symptoms by taking her medication with her to school and waiting until lunchtime to take them so she could continue with her classes.

Lingering Eye Problems

Even though some of the vision problems experienced by survivors after their discharge improved after a few weeks, eye-related problems continue to be a substantial health concern among survivors. The fact that temporary blindness was sometimes reversed with medication did not mean that the recovered patients were able to return to the same level of vision they had before. Indeed, among Ebola survivors a significant diversity of ocular (eye) problems has been found, ranging from occasional itching to complete blindness. Moreover, for many survivors, the problems with their eyesight started after they returned home from ETUs.

One such survivor was Kumba, a nurse at one of the largest hospitals in Freetown. While her ocular problems began after she was discharged, one aspect of her experiences was different from those found in other accounts. After she became infected with Ebola, she was admitted to what was then the most advanced treatment center in the country. It was a well-equipped ETU built and staffed by the British to provide care for Ebola-infected health care personnel. Given the fact that she received such an advanced level of care, it is unlikely that her complications were caused by a general lack of appropriate care available to Ebola patients at the time.

One morning after she returned home, Kumba woke up to realize that everything she saw was foggy. The problem lasted for several hours, so she went to an eye clinic to have it checked out. The initial treatment prescribed for her did not work. As a result, her eye problem deteriorated to the point that she almost lost vision in her right eye. During this period, she needed someone to hold onto as she walked and feared that she was about to become completely blind. Fortunately, the problem was addressed after additional medical treatment improved her vision. Yet her vision was never fully restored. As a result, she now needs reading glasses. As she described these experiences, she said one more thing that put her complications in perspective "But before, I did not have a problem with my eye. It was after I got sick that it started."

Estimates indicate that eye problems among Ebola survivors are very high. For example, uveitis (inflammation of the middle layer of the eye), the most common ocular complication observed among those infected with the disease, affects approximately 40% of all survivors.[12] Survivors have also been found to have other major eye complications, such as retina scarring and cataracts.[13] The most serious ocular complication found among them is complete loss of vision, which now requires those affected to adapt to the realities of being blind. Other survivors continue to have relatively milder eye-related problems, like near- or far-sightedness. For example, one survivor said, "If things are far away, I will see them a little bit better; closer to me, I will really not see them." The problem made it difficult for her to read. Although she was able to get prescription glasses from the hospital, she explained, "I still have a problem with my eyes because I always feel sharp pain in my eyes."

Apart from such pains, various symptoms of ocular problems were captured in the descriptions survivors gave of their ailments. Some of these include "My eyes become red, just like a fire"; [I feel like] "dew is in my eyes"; "my eyes are usually itching"; "my eyes really hurt"; "my eye is dim"; and "cataract grew over my eyes." In one case, a survivor described what he felt as a burning sensation in his eye so intense that he usually needed to "close [his] eyes for ten minutes" to get some sort of relief.

Other accounts indicated that the severity of these symptoms was higher at specific times of day. Accordingly, a few survivors mentioned that these symptoms were more severe around midday when they were directly under the sun. As one maintained, "When the sun is up and it is hot, my vision becomes dim, and I can't see properly except after sundown, that's when the problem goes away." This quote suggests that his eyes were sensitive to light, which is one of the many symptoms of uveitis.[14] In other cases, the symptoms were more substantial in the morning while survivors were trying to adjust to the first light of day.

Managing ocular complications was done concurrently with the task of managing other health and socioeconomic challenges. The best example that underscored this point was the case of Musu. She was the Ebola widow we met in chapter 3, who said she now served as the mother, father, and uncle to her five sons. She adjusted to these realities of widowhood while also dealing with eye complications she described as follows:

My eyes really give me a hard time. Sometimes it seems like something has come over my eyes like plastic. It's like when you are peeling an egg. There is that thin skin that covers the egg. Sometimes I feel like the same thing has come over my eyes. I even went to [the hospital] and the people gave me eye-drops, which I use. When I put them in my eyes, they itch, tears are usually running down my eyes.

These sequelae were only part of Musu's challenges because she also had frequent joint pains in her leg. She used to receive care for these issues through the free services provided by an international organization. However, her health problems continued. As a result, she was now raising five sons with restricted mobility due to joint pains while at the same time dealing with eye-related problems that made her situation more complex.

Most of the instrumental consequences of these ocular problems were those that negatively affected survivors' overall quality of life. They include the challenges faced by students who already faced difficulties readjusting to life in the classroom. Because these complications negatively affected their vision, many of them found it hard to study. Outside classroom contexts, eye complications negatively affected labor force participation. One example was found in the experiences of someone who previously worked as a tailor but was now unemployed due to his limited vision. More generally, the most tragic account of these issues was provided by a survivor describing the broader impacts of ocular problems on the lives of his counterparts. One of his peers with vision problems attempted to travel alone on a known footpath in a nearby forest. He subsequently went missing while attempting to do this. A few days later, his corpse was found in another area of the forest, which led him to believe that his friend died after he became lost due to his worsened vision.

These were only some of the many consequences of the ocular problems found among Ebola survivors in the study. Another included blindness, which is associated with highly complex physiological and social consequences. However, no blind survivor was interviewed for the study, although there are extensive reports of blind Ebola survivors in the affected countries. For the most part, blindness among them was caused by damage to the retina and optic nerve that went untreated over a long period.[15] Estimates indicate that in Sierra Leone alone, as many as a thousand Ebola survivors who have now completely lost their vision.[16] The problem has been documented among the elderly and survivors as young as five years old.[17]

Corresponding patterns have also been observed in the prevalence of cataracts, usually found among the elderly but now becoming a serious problem among children.[18] Significantly, the high prevalence of blindness and cataracts among survivors who are children raises the probability that some Ebola orphans may be affected. If this is correct, it would add to the other challenges they encounter in their everyday lives as they attempt to recover. Experiences of blindness have also been widely documented among survivors in Liberia. Like their counterparts in Sierra Leone, many Liberian survivors suffer from untreated eye-related problems that can lead to blindness.[19]

The Chronic Pain of Musculoskeletal Disorders

Five members of Momo's family died within one week, which was among the most dramatic things he recalled about the spread of the virus during the epidemic in Liberia. After they died, the rest of his family was taken to various ETUs, where they were diagnosed with Ebola virus disease. Fortunately, Momo was one of four people in the family who survived. However, his stay at the ETU where he was admitted was relatively long—about eight weeks. Among the things he recalled about his time there was the problem he had with diarrhea, which became so bad that blood began to show up in his stools. Another was the accumulation of dead bodies—naked bodies of people who looked like they were as old as his parents.

Since returning home from the ETU, his recovery process has been filled with new problems. He experiences what he refers to as traumas driven by the flashbacks he regularly has of his time at the ETU. In addition, he suffered from temporary leg problems that left him unable to walk by himself; he subsequently recovered from this disability. Perhaps because of this experience, he now lives with chronic sharp back pains. Unfortunately, none of the medication he has received has helped to alleviate the problem. As a result, he has drawn the following conclusion: "I have decided to live with it. Only God knows why this is happening."

Musculoskeletal disorders, or problems related to the injury of muscles, joints, nerves, and tendons, represent another common health complication found among Ebola survivors. Some of these complications are temporal, like Momo's experience of becoming physically disabled; however, like his back pains, most are chronic. Shortly after the end of the epidemic, one study of survivors in Montserrado county in Monrovia found that within three months after Ebola survivors' recovery, about 77% experienced joint pain, 68% muscle pain, and 67% chest pain.[20] A similar study conducted among survivors from an ETU at the 34 Military Hospital in Sierra Leone found that 70% suffered from musculoskeletal problems.[21] In general, the prevalence of these problems declines over time, with one study suggesting that it drops to less than 10% after a few years.[22] Still, the problems associated with musculoskeletal complications and their corresponding pains are ongoing issues that continue to affect the lives of survivors.

Among the many ways this occurs is by creating new physical disabilities that adversely affect survivors' quality of life. Like Momo, many survivors have effectively decided to "live with" chronic pains. However, this uncomfortable process limits their capacity to support themselves and requires the development of adaptive behaviors. The sources of these disabilities are diverse. For one, they include the many side effects of survivors' medical treatments received while in ETUs. Years later, survivors continue to feel pain in parts of their bodies where intravenous needles were inserted. Other pains are due to complications that have led to inflammation in their joints, abdominal pain, and numbness in various parts of their bodies. At first, these pains can be confusing because they are quite similar to many of those experienced as the early symptoms of Ebola infection. This usually added to the plethora of factors that fueled doubts about whether survivors were still infected with the disease.

Some of the ways in which these disorders shaped survivors' everyday experiences were captured in an account provided by Lucy, who lived in Monrovia's Montserrado County, and whose musculoskeletal disorders occurred along with other comorbidities. Her main musculoskeletal ailment was numbness in her hands, possibly due to nerve injury, as well as chronic pains in her hands and knees. These maladies had not responded to treatment with medication. As a result, she developed several adaptive behaviors to help her live with them, to reduce the negative toll they had on her quality of life. As she explained:

> Right now, as I am talking to you, my head is spinning . . . my hands get numb. Anything that I am doing, like washing myself up, braiding hair or even using a pen to write, anything I am doing will just get my hands numb. My hands get

numb even when I am sleeping. The pain wakes me up in the middle part of the night. I am taking medication, but it is still not helping, and it is really embarrassing. At times, when I am washing myself up, my hands get numb, then I have to wait for minutes and squeeze them, like I am praying, before the numbness ends, then I start washing again. And my knee, now I can't really like stand properly when I wake up, I have to struggle before I stand up straight.

Of all the musculoskeletal disorders observed among Ebola survivors, the one most frequently experienced by those interviewed in the study was chronic joint pains. These pains were not just restricted to the hands and knees. It extended to their necks, elbows, backs, and other parts of their bodies. The pains were described as severe, constant, and feeling like both hands and knees were "tied together." One survivor said, "When I lie down, I am tormented." Regardless of where joint pains occurred, their consequences were the same in the sense that they limited survivors' ability to perform tasks they used to be able to do.

For example, when asked whether she continues to experience the symptoms of the illness she had during the first month of recovery, one Sierra Leonean survivor responded as follows:

> Yes, the pains. I can't bend down to wash my clothes. My foot also hurts. I can't lay it down while sleeping. When I raise it up I feel less pain. I can't stand up for a long time nor can I sit down for a long time. I have to raise it up. Sometimes I can't get up for days. I also feel pain in the muscle in the leg. I can't do small household chores until the pain subsides. Only Allah can make this go away.

Another survivor, who was also dealing with ocular problems, combined her experience with these issues with those associated with frequent pain in her foot. She had a unique way of putting the latter perspective that involved describing what was about to happen at the end of the interview. She said, "Right now, after sitting down for this interview, when I try to stand up again, it is going to be difficult . . . I still get a lot of joint pains." Much of the pain was concentrated in her left foot. The pains were so severe that she could no longer walk for long distances as she did before she was infected with Ebola.

Other survivors talked about their experiences with chronic pains that limited their ability to do simple things such as lifting buckets of water or performing their jobs. In some cases, the pains are cyclical; that is, they vary depending on seasonal temperature changes. For example, low temperatures that started with the onset of the rainy season made joint pains worse. In the Susan's Bay slum community in Freetown, for example, this relationship between low temperatures and chronic pain had a particularly negative effect on the work of a fisherman who was a survivor. Because it is usually cold at sea, the pain makes it difficult for him to do his job. Another survivor in the same community mentioned that it is so intense that she has to stay home from work when the pain starts. When this occurs, her family depends on her neighbors for sustenance, which they usually provide by sharing their food, since her husband was unemployed.

Other Health Problems

Ebola survivors lived with other health complications that cannot be fully described here due to space limitations. None of them was as prevalent as the mental, ocular, and musculoskeletal health issues reviewed above, but this does not mean they are less significant. Part of this group of other complications are sexual and reproductive health issues. Often more highly prevalent among females than males, these issues adversely affected their physiological, psychological, and social well-being.

Girls and women with reproductive health issues were most likely to have menstrual cycles that had either become irregular or completely ceased. Estimates indicate that the problem is experienced by 5% to 11% of all female survivors.[23] However, the clinical reasons for the problem are unclear. Some scholars suggest that it is among the many serious health complications found among survivors with a high viral load when infected.[24] No viral load information was available for survivors interviewed for the study. Therefore, it is impossible to make direct inferences about its association with variations in the symptoms reported by girls and women. At the same time, there were variations in these experiences that were difficult to ignore. For example, some cases of menstrual cessation were permanent, while others were temporary. One survivor reported that she did not menstruate for nine months after being discharged but that her menstrual cycle resumed after receiving treatment from the hospital.

As a result of these menstrual problems, a few female survivors mentioned that they had been unable to conceive. Among this group, the perception of a positive association between Ebola infection and infertility was most salient among those who had given birth before the epidemic but have not been able to get pregnant again. Reports suggest that childbearing problems of female survivors may be extensive. Shortly after the end of the epidemic, for example, research indicated that female survivors had disproportionately higher rates of stillbirths.[25] Thus, female Ebola survivors appear to have had problems with both conceiving and delivering live births. These issues are particularly concerning because most West African societies place a high premium on women's ability to have children. Therefore, problems with infertility could create a source of social tension between female survivors and members of their community, which could affect how well they are integrated into social life.

Male survivors experienced sexual health issues that were primarily driven by various forms of erectile dysfunction. Their accounts described two aspects of the problem. The first was the perception that their erections were not as firm as they were before. The second was associated with difficulties they experienced with becoming aroused. Both of these negatively affected their ability to experience sexual pleasure. Additionally, they had psychological consequences. In particular, they affected the men's sense of pride because of implicit questions they raised about their manhood. To make this point, one survivor disclosed that the period after the epidemic was the first time he had a sexual experience with a female partner who asked him whether he was "finished" while they were still having sex. The question left him feeling particularly embarrassed because it was asked while he was finding it difficult to ejaculate.

A final set of complications were a diverse collection of ailments such as ulcers, dermatological problems, and miscellaneous issues that were difficult to classify. The few individuals who said they had had frequent ulcers also reported occasional stomach pains. However, it was difficult to confirm whether there was a connection between the two since stomach pains could result from either peptic ulcers or musculoskeletal disorders. Other problems included extensive skin exfoliation and reported hot sensations under the feet. Additionally, one female survivor indicated that she had not been able to stoop down to pee. As a result, she now consistently stands up when using the bathroom. This symptom was concerning, but the clinical reasons for it were unclear.

Institutional Responses to the Health of Survivors

Ebola survivors continue to deal with all these health complications, despite the fact that medical treatments are available to manage many of them effectively. Steroid therapy can be used to reverse some forms of blindness,[26] while cataract surgery can improve vision. With the help of psychiatrists and other mental health professionals, many mental health conditions can also be effectively managed, while other health complications can similarly be ameliorated with appropriate medical care. Although all these treatment options are available in countries with modern health systems, the health systems of Liberia and Sierra Leone are anything but modern.

In view of these lingering problems survivors have with the sequalae of Ebola, it is important to answer the following question: How have local health institutions responded to address these issues? The short answer is that their responses have been inadequate. Although this answer is correct, it needs to be put in perspective. For starters, the capacity of health institutions to respond to these issues has been undermined by the epidemic due to the death of health care personnel. Before then, decades of underinvestment in health care meant that both Liberia and Sierra Leone were medical deserts, and to a large extent, things remain the same.[27]

Despite these similarities, however, there is a notable difference in the response of health care institutions in both countries. Overall, the response to the ongoing needs of survivors has been stronger in Liberia than in Sierra Leone. This response does not imply that survivors are receiving comprehensive health care in the former. They are not. In fact, in both countries, a more comprehensive response to the health care essentials of survivors is needed. This response should prioritize programs that address the social factors that negatively affect access to the health care needed for tackling the medical consequences of the epidemic. In the months following the end of the epidemic, survivors in both countries had free access to medical care.

Since then, Liberia has provided a slightly better level of access to health care for survivors than Sierra Leone. Much of this has occurred through the Partnership for Research on Vaccines and Infectious Disease programs in Liberia (PREVAIL). Mainly located at JFK Hospital in Monrovia, PREVAIL was formed as a partnership between Liberia's Ministry of Health and the U.S. National Institutes of Health. It provides Ebola survivors access to essential health care services, which are mostly linked with participation in the two institutions' clinical studies on mental health and vision problems.

When Liberian survivors mentioned that they had received eyedrops, blood tests, or procedures recently, they were mostly referring to the services given during their visits to the facilities of PREVAIL. This does not mean that the care they received from PREVAIL was perfect; a few survivors had concerns about the treatment they were receiving from PREVAIL.[28] Despite their worries, there was no question that a centralized structure was available in Liberia to address their health complications, that the treatment they received was free, and that the services provided have generally continued to be available since the end of the epidemic.

Across the border in Sierra Leone, the institutional response has been comparatively weaker. Free medical care was initially provided to survivors by either NGOs or the Connaught Hospital, which is the main government hospital in the country, during the epidemic. However, survivors' access to these services ended about two years after the epidemic, leaving them without any real access to modern health care. This unfortunate transition coincided with two developments. The first was the scaling down of the operations of NGOs at the end of the epidemic, which effectively curtailed their partnership with the government to provide medical services. The second was a change in government administration. Among survivors, this change is considered to have led to a shift from an administration that played an active role in promoting their welfare to one that had no commitment to do so.

Under these circumstances, it was not surprising that declines in access to health care were among the many problems raised by a leader of the national Ebola survivors' association while discussing the challenges faced by his members. He started by focusing on the positive role played by NGOs just after the end of the epidemic. In the process, he created the following picture of the previous system, which addressed most of the health care needs of survivors:

One of the positive ways NGOs helped survivors was found in a project implemented by the government, in collaboration with other organizations such as

UKAID, Partners in Health, and IMC-Go Sierra Leone. They created a medical . . . health program for survivors, that allowed survivors to visit the hospital, while other survivors served as health advocates, which made the medical situation more effective. At that time, these programs were also being monitored effectively.

When asked to compare the assistance they received then with what is currently available to Ebola survivors, he responded:

> Really, back then, the assistance was good, it was great, it was encouraging, but currently things have declined. There is no help now, no way now, no doors you can knock on. So, people are stranded. They are worse off now; they are suffering, complications have been increasing; health complications, hunger, illiteracy, you know, a lot of people are now worse off. No more help is coming from organizations like before. No assistance is being consistently provided to us now compared to the past. Nothing is going on with the free medical care that the government promised us. When Ebola survivors go to the hospital, they are marginalized, they are stigmatized. No one pays attention to them, so they have to find money to take care of themselves.

Patterns of Health-Seeking Behavior Among Ebola Survivors

With no regular access to health care, survivors have found other ways to deal with the various medical conditions they continue to experience. However, the process of choosing to address these conditions is complicated by the fact that many of the survivors were already part of the marginalized poor before the epidemic. Nowhere else were these complications more evident than in the western part of Moyamba district in Sierra Leone, home of the only rural survivors interviewed for the study.

These individuals mostly lived in the vicinity of Bradford, near an area where the virus was reported to have spread after a health care worker unknowingly transmitted it to his patients. Survivors in the area face many of the same health challenges faced by their counterparts in Freetown and Monrovia. Nevertheless, when asked whether they had seen a doctor during the past year, the nature of their response was captured in replies provided by two individuals. The first was a female survivor who said, "No, because it is expensive. If I go, I will not be able to take care of my family and get us something to eat." The second was another female survivor who expressed the same idea, with the following deflection: "We don't even have food. I have to go and beg for rice to cook before my family can eat." This response indicated that feeding her family was more important than paying to see a doctor.

Similar reactions were observed among Ebola survivors in Freetown, even though they lived in slightly better socioeconomic circumstances. Many of them observed that since the end of the policy of free access to health care, visiting a doctor had become very expensive. As a result, the difficulties they now encountered with getting access to medical care were the same as those they faced before the epidemic. As one of them put it, "If you don't go with money, no one looks at you, even if you show them your certificate indicating that you are an Ebola survivor. No one looks at you."

Treatment for their many health complications is now secured through two strategies of health-seeking behavior. The first is the use of traditional African medicine, which is used either by itself or in combination with the minimal modern health care available to those who can afford it. Traditional medicine in Africa is sometimes misunderstood by people who imply that it is based more on myth than on science. In fairness, some of these criticisms are correct, given the many limitations of traditional medicine. In fact, one reason for the rapid spread of Ebola in the early part of the epidemic was the belief by infected persons in Liberia, Guinea, and Sierra Leone that the disease could be cured using traditional medicine.[29] However, there is a long history of using traditional herbs, oils, and other organic materials to help individuals recover from ailments in African societies.

These practices are now seen as useful alternatives to modern health care. One survivor, for example, said that he treated his persistent joint pains by using what he referred to as "country medicine." He described it as traditional herbs, which were "bought by [his] wife to apply on [him], as well as crushed ginger to rub on to [his] bones for [his body] to become strong." For another survivor, the preferred solution for similar pains was to "boil native medicine" so that the liquid solution could be used during a shower to warm his body. Another use of "native medicine" was to wash the eyes of those with vision problems to enable them to see clearly. There was just one problem with such uses of traditional medicine. All those who admitted to using them continued to experience the very same symptoms they were attempting to address. At the same time, this use of traditional medicine underscored a crucial point. Left with little to no afford-able source of modern health care, survivors have been willing to try other options that may not be effective.

The second strategy used by survivors was self-medication using modern Western medicine. This strategy typically involved purchasing over-the-counter drugs from regular pharmacies or drug peddlers on the street. The latter are particularly problematic because they sometimes sell over-the-counter and prescription drugs of questionable origins while occasionally providing dubious medical advice. The main health conditions self-medication addressed were those related to chronic pain. Furthermore, survivors engaged in this behavior more widely after the policy of free access to medical care for survivors was discontinued. Apart from the fact that it has inherent risks, self-medication was probably not very effective because it is used less frequently when survivors run out of money. More importantly, even when it temporarily helped to ease their symptoms, it did not address the underlying causes of their complications. Perhaps this was one reason why many self-medicating survivors continued to experience the various symptoms associated with their health complications.

Complications of Ebola and Social Consequences of the Epidemic

All this occurred on the heels of the extensive international response observed during the 2014 Ebola epidemic. It paved the way for what was arguably one of the most successful international interventions recently mounted to stop the spread of a deadly virus. The scale of medical resources committed to this endeavor was significant. It drew on the expertise of some of the world's best epidemiologists, physicians, and other health personnel as well as the resources of some of the world's well-funded humanitarian organizations. Nevertheless, the success of the global effort was quickly followed by the withdrawal of these resources at the end of the epidemic. Limited attempts were made to invest in the failing health systems that were partly responsible for the crisis, and no long-term strategy was developed for addressing the future health complications that survivors would experience. These complications were predictable because the sequelae of infection with the virus had been extensively documented during previous outbreaks.

This failure to transition from relief to development left the affected countries in the same health care situation they were in before the start of the epidemic. Failure to invest in their health systems left them incapable of providing essential treatments and specialized services to address the ensuing health problems. For example, Sierra Leone continues to have only five ophthalmology consultants in the whole country to provide specialized services for eye problems.[30] Additionally, it has 2 psychiatrists, 2 clinical psychologists, and 19 mental health nurses for its population of about 7 million people.[31] Liberia is no less disadvantaged. Despite the fact that it provides more consistent services to survivors than Sierra Leone, estimates indicate that it has only two psychiatrists to address the mental health needs of its population of about five million.[32]

Meanwhile, many Ebola survivors continue to live with chronic conditions that have had far-reaching implications for their quality of life. These conditions have negatively affected their ability to resume basic daily activities such as taking a shower, reading, and sleeping uninterrupted. At the same time, they have contributed to the subjection of survivors to the social indignities experienced by people believed to be insane, infertile, or unable to have healthy sexual relationships. For these reasons, the return of survivors to their communities has been accompanied by substantial decreases in their ability to live independently and participate in the life of their communities. Much of this could have been avoided by making the investments needed to increase their access to health care. However, these investments have been lacking because of the limited attention given to the consequences of the epidemic.

5   The Stickiness of Stigma

Kumba learned a key lesson after she returned to work following her recovery from Ebola: Even within the health care field, survivors are not immune from the stigma associated with the disease. As a nurse working in Freetown, her experience with such stigma started long before she contracted the virus. It began when she was assigned to the outpatient unit of one of the city's largest hospitals during the epidemic. At that time, she began to notice that nurses in other units were treating her with an unusual sense of suspicion. This was because the outpatient unit was the first place in the hospital where patients who might have Ebola were treated. Caring for these patients led other nurses to believe that Kumba was already contagious, but this was not true. Subsequently, however, she became infected with Ebola and was transferred to an ETU, where she remained until she was discharged. Kumba's return to work increased her encounters with stigma now that others knew that she had, indeed, been infected.

What was surprising about the stigmatization she experienced was the fact that it occurred in the health care sector—among people who should know that Ebola survivors are no longer contagious after testing negative for the virus. However, this was not an isolated event. Many health care workers in West Africa faced similar types of stigmatization after they recovered from Ebola. This did not mean they did not have colleagues who reacted positively to them after they returned. What was clear was that these positive responses did not preclude survivors from experiencing prejudice, ostracization, and rejection at institutions where few would expect such experiences to occur.

Encounters with stigma experienced by nurses were possibly a small fraction of the prejudice observed among survivors during the epidemic.

During this period, close to 63% of survivors in Liberia were stigmatized,[1] while 54.8% of those in Sierra Leone experienced at least one encounter with stigma.[2] These negative encounters were so pervasive that they affected survivors' interactions with others, their psychosocial wellbeing, and their ability to reintegrate into their communities. What's more, the stigma of Ebola was difficult to eradicate. In fact, it continues to be a significant factor that affects the social lives of survivors. This enduring character of the stigma of Ebola is important and is a major factor that distinguishes the social consequences of the Ebola epidemic from those associated with other diseases.

Very little is known about the "stickiness" of the stigma observed in recent epidemics, such as those associated with COVID-19, bird flu, or the Zika virus. However, what is known about the stigma observed during these crises suggests that they differ from the stigma of Ebola in several ways. First, the stigma of these other diseases is mostly experienced by individuals in marginalized populations, such as racial and ethnic minorities. A clear example of this was the selective targeting of individuals for stigmatization during the COVID-19 epidemic in the United States. Accordingly, Asian immigrants and other racial/ethnic minorities who were suspected of being carriers of the disease were subject to scorn, ridicule, and other negative responses from people in their communities.[3] By contrast, among the many millions of people who had COVID-19 and subsequently recovered, experiences with stigma were rare, according to what recent estimates suggest.[4]

Second, the stigma of Ebola lingers in distinctive ways that negatively affect the social lives of survivors, the places where they live, and the lives of their loved ones. Perhaps due to the intense fear of the high mortality rate of the disease, many survivors continue to be seen as potential threats long after their recovery. In some cases, Ebola infections have been associated with high levels of stigma that remain stable for up to a year after patients have recovered.[5] While the overall prevalence of Ebola-related stigma subsequently declines, the stigma of disease is all too often invoked to discriminate against those who had the disease several years after their recovery.

Among the various consequences of the Ebola epidemic itself, stigma also stands out in other important ways. Consider that the consequences associated with the health complications of the disease and the lost livelihoods of survivors can be addressed by directly providing resources to ameliorate these burdens. In contrast, the problems associated with stigma are not as amenable to these types of investments, and the reasons for this are diverse. For one, the source of the problem targeted by health investments is in the physical bodies of survivors, whereas the source of the stigma problem lies not with survivors but with others in their communities. This does not imply that there are no implications of stigma for the physical well-being of survivors. Rather, it underscores the fact that the investments needed to address the consequences of stigma at the individual level are less effective for addressing the source of the problem compared to investments that address the true source of the problem, which is found at the level of communities.

Perhaps for these reasons, policy interest in tackling the problem of stigma is less institutionalized compared to policy interest in other social domains. While specialized agencies such as the United Nations Development Program and the United Nations Children's Fund exist to tackle the latter, none of the well-known international development agencies focuses on the problem of stigma. Therefore, it is not surprising that the range of post-epidemic interventions used to address the lingering consequences of Ebola stigma has been small. As such, more will need to be done to ameliorate these consequences using carefully crafted social responses. Owing to their high levels of effectiveness, social inventions targeting the stigma problem have been used extensively in previous epidemics to improve relationships between victims and members of their communities. Some of the most notable of these were visible in the anti-stigma campaigns at the height of the HIV/AIDS crisis in countries such as South Africa, Uganda, and the United States in recent decades.[6]

Social programs addressing stigma in local communities were used on a comparatively limited scale by aid organizations in West Africa in the aftermath of the Ebola epidemic.[7] These efforts were not on par with the multiyear campaigns used to address during the HIV/AIDS epidemic. Instead, they were short-term programs, which had some level of success but were incapable of comprehensively tackling the complexities of the stigma of Ebola. These complexities were significant and rooted in cultural narratives about the nature of disease, community fears about its association with death, and existing patterns of social class disadvantage. Unfortunately, there are no obvious solutions to address the issues created by these complexities. As a result, the problem of stigma continues to be an intractable one that has continued to affect the lives of many survivors since the end of the epidemic.

Developing a portrait of these complexities requires paying careful attention to several important issues. Central to these is the question of why patients who had been confirmed as testing negative for the virus continued to be viewed as threats to their community after they were discharged. To answer this question, it is vital to understand how residents in these communities attempted to reconcile what they had been told about the virus with the realities they faced when meeting people they knew had been infected with Ebola before. Also important is the need for a careful examination of how stigma affected, and continues to affect, the day-to-day experiences of survivors. These consequences of stigma operate through microsocial processes that affect survivors' relationships with their neighbors, coworkers, and others who play important roles within the social fabric of their communities.

Although the impacts of stigma on these relationships are significant, they need to be juxtaposed with an understanding of the various attempts made to mitigate their consequences. These mitigation strategies are extensive, and as will be discussed shortly, they were seen in the interventions developed by various actors such as NGOs, community leaders, and Ebola survivors themselves. On the basis of these interventions, a useful set of strategies can be identified for developing long-term solutions to the problems posed by stigma.

Fear, Ebola Prevention, and the Development of Stigma

Very few communities just decide to stigmatize their own residents without the influence of outside social forces. For those receiving Ebola survivors returning from ETUs, the primary force was the fear of the disease. This fear thrived in an environment that was muddled by the confusing messages that were found in Ebola prevention campaigns. In addition, it was difficult for locals to reconcile the apparent contradictions found in what they had been told about the virus. On the one hand, messages of prevention had emphasized that Ebola was a deadly disease that had no cure. On the other hand, the people they knew had been infected with the virus were now returning home, claiming to be healed. This disparity between what they had been told and what survivors were saying was substantial. As such, the key question that many neighbors asked survivors after they returned home was this: "How can you claim you no longer have Ebola when we have been told that it has no cure?" From their neighbors' perspective, only a few answers to this question were considered acceptable. Among them was the fact that those claiming to be survivors were either bewitched, liars, or part of the walking dead.[8]

Things were further complicated by the need to deal with two additional realities. Ebola prevention campaigns had also provided a list of symptoms that were useful for identifying people who were potentially contagious. These included redness of the eye, vomiting, body aches, and abdominal pains. However, these were among the same symptoms that survivors continued to experience as they struggled with complications in the weeks following their discharge. Based on the information they had at the time, locals who saw gaunt-looking survivors, with eyes that were red from ocular complications, took the easy road by becoming risk averse. For them, ostracizing Ebola survivors who were now returning to their communities was a rational reaction created by the need for self-preservation.

Some NGO representatives who worked in West Africa during the epidemic now acknowledge that, while well intentioned, many aspects of the messaging of anti-Ebola campaigns were responsible for the stigmatization of survivors.[9] Public messages that admonished people to avoid touching those with suspected symptoms had been designed with very little nuance. As such, it was not always easy to determine how to put these messages into practice when dealing with persons who had now been determined to be Ebola-free. With widespread knowledge of the high mortality risks associated with Ebola, therefore, the path of least resistance involved using the fear of the disease as a central axis that determined social relations.

Survivors' first experiences with these new social relations occurred on the day they arrived home. At that point, their exposure to stigma was usually tempered by an interplay of emotions involving fear, happiness, and curiosity. Those who still had living relatives were received by people caught between the desire to respond and the conflicting demands of these emotions. Some relatives had believed rumors about the death of their loved ones in ETUs and had already started the process of mourning. However, the mourning process was often interrupted by the delight they felt by receiving their kin alive. Most of these celebrations were short-lived due to lingering concerns about whether survivors were still contagious. In the larger communities that survivors were returning to, such celebrations were rare. More common were the burning concerns about the presence of people most residents considered to still be contagious.

Community Fears and the Stigmatization of Survivors

Yeabu's recollection of the day she was discharged began by observing that her young baby and herself were the only 2 individuals who survived out of the more than 20 people in her household who had contracted the virus. She returned to her close-knit rural community on the outskirts of Freetown, contemplating what the future would hold without her father and grandparents, who were her main sources of support. As if this burden was not enough, she observed something remarkably different about the neighbors who were around when she returned. None of them tried to approach her; in fact, not one of them tried to embrace her. This was not a reflection of their ambivalence toward Yeabu's return. Instead, it was an indication of the negative reactions they had toward her, which later became obvious when she attempted to visit their home. On the day of her visit, the neighbors were sitting outside in their yard. However, when they saw her walking toward them, they simply got up and left, letting her know of their disapproval and that her presence there was not welcomed.

Yeabu's experience with stigma increased in subsequent weeks, when her neighbors stopped allowing her to use the shortcut to the local market that passed through their compounds. She was denied access to a well that was located at a nearby house by the owner pretending she had lost the gate key to prevent her from entering the compound. Other neighbors, with whom she used to share her meals, no longer wanted to eat what she had cooked.

Although she had suspicions about why her neighbors were now acting differently, it was what she heard someone say about her and her child that confirmed these suspicions. The confirmation came in the form of a warning she heard one of them give to other locals about her and her child: "They are Ebola survivors. You need to be careful around them." After this experience, Yeabu decided to keep to herself, isolating herself and her baby from the rest of her community.

Unlike the living relatives receiving survivors returning home from ETUs, the broader community had less of an incentive to resume relationships with these survivors. Their neighbors were not as emotionally invested in these relationships compared to their relatives, and, as observed in chapter 3, even relatives who were supposed to have these emotional investments were now apprehensive about resuming these relationships. Notably, the fear of contagion was reason enough for people to distance themselves from survivors, and this type of ostracizing is precisely what stigma is designed to do. Goffman, in his classic discussion of stigma, argues that it is an attribute designed to "reduce the bearer from a whole or usual person to a tainted, discounted one."[10] Consequently, people who are believed to be bearers of such tainted attributes become easy targets for discrimination, labeling, and the loss of social status.[11]

Such responses would not have mattered if the lives of survivors and their community members were not so intertwined in bonds of mutual dependence. These bonds were critical for gaining access to resources, developing friendships, and participating in everyday activities, things that were central to community life. In normal circumstances, the stability of these relationships would have provided a useful foundation from which survivors could expect to begin the process of rebuilding their lives. However, these were not normal circumstances. As a result, many of these social bonds were destroyed due to the stigma surrounding Ebola, which fractured the foundations of community life in ways that upended survivors' expectations. Breaks in these relationships made it difficult for them to do mundane tasks, such as sharing meals, traveling, or having casual conversations. By creating these new obstacles to social reintegration, the stigma of Ebola imposed new burdens on survivors and undermined their status as productive members of society.

The practical challenges created by this stigma were generally observed across borders. One survivor in Liberia, for example, noted how hiring an *okada* (a motorbike taxi), a cheap means of local transportation, became a problem for him because no one wanted to touch survivors. This occurred at a time when he had just started to experience some of the long-term complications of Ebola and was unable to walk long distances. Reports from interviews conducted in both Liberia and Sierra Leone, which are predominantly rural societies, further indicate that the negative effect of stigma on survivors' ability to fetch water from community wells was a very common problem. Other experiences of stigma were somewhat rare. They included an account of being prevented from dumping trash at the local trash dump, presumably because the trash of survivors was considered to be contagious. Another example was an account of a survivor who was asked to move to a building where chickens were kept, instead of into the main house, as a way of keeping them away from house residents.

A larger issue that survivors had to confront was the question of whether locals, in fact, wanted their very presence in the community. Some locals who did not used subtle clues to express this, including their refusal to provide services to survivors or allow them to participate in community activities. Others were more direct and communicated their disdain for survivors by being more explicit in their deployment of stigma.

This more explicit response was what a man selling sneakers in Montserrado county in Liberia captured in his recollection of his experiences with stigma. He was a well-known resident of his community before his infection. However, after being discharged, he decided to spend some time with his parents in another community before returning to his apartment. Although no one in his parents' community stigmatized him when he returned to his apartment, his neighbors expressed their outrage at his presence in the community. They made it clear that his presence was unwelcome and justified their anger by saying that his return was premature. Their preference was for him to stay away from the neighborhood until *they* were convinced that he had recovered from the disease.

Underlying this response was another stigma-related problem that survivors encountered after being discharged—the problem of finding suitable accommodation. Presumed to be tainted by Ebola, survivors faced the discriminatory actions of neighbors and landlords who refused to allow them to live in their midst as a way of keeping them at a distance. For example, a survivor in Liberia maintained that her neighbors did not allow her live-in boyfriend and herself to return to their house because, as she put it, "They did not want me to be carrying the virus in their community." As a result, they left and went to live with her brother and his wife.

Landlords wielded more power to prevent survivors from living in their midst because they had a more effective tool—the power to evict—at their disposal to enforce their discrimination. Some of their decisions to evict survivors flew in the face of reason. One case in point was that of someone who lived in Kakata, Liberia, when she was discharged, and like many other survivors, had received a certificate from an ETU indicating that she had indeed tested negative for Ebola. When she arrived home, however, she discovered that her landlord had already decided to ask her to leave. Nothing she did changed his mind, including presenting him with the certificate she had received from the ETU. Instead, she recalled, "He told me, 'You can't live in this house right now, because you are an Ebola survivor.' So, I said 'Oh, you should be happy for me since you did not hear that I had died. God made me survive. But, even though I came back, you are saying that I can't live in the house.'"

Landlords in Sierra Leone were not necessarily different from those in Liberia. As one survivor in Freetown recounted, her landlord decided to evict her even after she had paid her monthly rent in full. Indeed, he was so concerned about avoiding physical contact with her that he requested that she collect her rent at a local police station, where he had asked an officer to hold it until she returned home. Other landlords indirectly pushed survivors out of their premises by substantially increasing rents. In many cases, the rent hikes were disguised to appear benign; however, it was occasionally possible to connect the dots to understand the underlying reasons why they were occurring. Another survivor thus reported that he had an encounter with his landlord's brother, who told him that he would never talk to him again because he was afraid of the disease. Shortly thereafter, he received notice from the landlord indicating that his rent had been increased to an amount he was now unable to afford.

Labeling, Stigma, and Encounters in Public Spaces

These examples highlight only some of the ways in which the social relationships that existed before the Ebola epidemic were fractured in its aftermath. At the same time, they underscore the contrast between the expectations that survivors had of their communities and the realities they faced after they returned. Speaking of the stigma she experienced with her siblings, for example, one survivor said, "I expected a lot from my community because no one gets an Ebola infection on purpose. We are not enemies."

As she continued to speak about her experiences, she revealed how another strategy, the use of labels, was used by her neighbors to identify her and other survivors as threats to the community. To illustrate, she began by discussing the details of how her mother's death from Ebola left her and her younger siblings with limited means to survive. Accordingly, she decided to initiate contact with a neighbor who owed her mother some money before she died. She sent one of her younger siblings to the person's home to ask for the debt to be repaid. However, her account of what happened when the sibling arrived is instructive:

> When my younger sister got there, someone who knew my mother saw her and started yelling, "This is an Ebola child. This is an Ebola child. She needs to leave this place." So, my sister returned home crying. As for me, I thank God because I was not paying that much attention to them. I just focused my mind on the new responsibilities I now had. People were afraid of me. They were not coming near us.

Unsurprisingly, this incident left her and her young sibling in tears. Most accounts survivors provided of their stigma experiences were followed by acknowledging subsequent feelings of sadness, as well as episodes of crying. These reactions are among what are now recognized as the implications of stigma for survivors' mental health. Along with feelings of shame and guilt, these symptoms are among the manifestations of the psychosocial consequences of Ebola infection.[12]

Labeling survivors as people who were still infected had other social consequences. Some of these were observed in a study conducted in Freetown that asked 24 children orphaned by Ebola to draw whatever came to mind when they thought about a child in a family affected by the virus.[13] In addition, they were requested to write from 3 to 10 phrases that explained the images they had drawn. By the end of the study, most of the children had drawn pictures showing how Ebola-orphaned children were ostracized. One image showed a picture of classmates pointing fingers at an orphan who had just returned to school. Another picture showed an orphan attempting to purchase food from a trader, only to see the trader refuse to accept his money. Particularly troubling was that the images also depicted adults using the pejorative label "Ebola child" to refer to orphans. Stigmatizing children in this way can significantly reduce the likelihood that they will turn to local adults when faced with emergencies.

At the same time, this stigmatization can affect the social lives of children by limiting interactions with their peers. Adult influences on their children partly drives this social isolation. Interviews in Liberia and Sierra Leone revealed multiple accounts of incidents in which children of survivors who were outside playing with other children saw parents of the latter call them home because of lingering fears of contagion. Older children had their own experiences of stigma, largely driven by the actions of their peer-group members. The primary examples of these were found in the accounts of survivors who attended school and reported being stigmatized by their friends and of child survivors with neighborhood peers who reconfigured their social activities to exclude friends whom they feared were contagious.

Another dimension of the resumption of the social lives of survivors involved moving beyond the walls of their neighborhoods. These movements were associated with renewed interactions with institutions and individuals who did not know about their prior infection. When this information became known, however, it triggered new encounters with stigma in public places such as offices and schools, which had a slightly different texture compared to the stigmatization experiences survivors had within their neighborhoods. Part of this difference occurred because, in public spaces, the source of stigma was not always in close social proximity to survivors. This was seen, for example, in an account provided by a teacher interviewed in rural Sierra Leone, who maintained that some parents of students at his school disenrolled their children after they learned that he was a survivor.

Health institutions provided one setting where public encounters were experienced. These encounters extended beyond the specific experiences of nurses such as Kumba, who were stigmatized by colleagues after they returned to work. They were seen in the responses of patients who refused to let nurses who had recovered from Ebola take their vital signs. Their refusal came from concern that the process involved direct physical interaction with the nurses, which would ostensibly increase their chances of being infected. The encounters were also seen in other interactions between survivors and health personnel they met during their visits to hospitals for post-recovery medical care. One survivor, who was also a nurse, recalled having such an experience at another health care institution when she went for an eye exam to address her ocular problems. Given her familiarity with the way things worked in health care settings, however, she reported her experience to a doctor in the facility, who intervened to halt the discrimination.

Positive Responses and Deceptive Declines in Stigma

Widespread concerns about the presumed threat posed by survivors did not usually mean that they were stigmatized by everyone in their social circles. Stigma is a consequence of deliberate decisions taken by people based on information they have on characteristics, traits, or attributes they consider to be undesirable. Therefore, the decision to stigmatize is based on a choice, and after Ebola survivors returned home, other people they met made a different choice by responding to them positively. These positive responses were generally rare, but when they occurred, they provided a sense of normalcy and a renewed faith in the traditional values of community support.

While discussing these interactions, some survivors mentioned the assistance they received from such supportive neighbors. These neighbors either found innovative ways to navigate their fears and offer help or took direct action to help, contrary to the narrative of fear. One such neighbor regularly provided food that helped nurture a survivor, still weak after returning home, until she became strong. It involved finding new ways to help that avoided direct physical interaction between people. Accordingly, the neighbor frequently dropped off meals at the front door of the survivors' house, which she ate until she was strong enough to fend for herself.

Other neighbors responded positively as a direct reaction to the negative way survivors were being treated. This response came in handy for one survivor who reported that, after she was discharged from the ETU with her children, some of her neighbors refused to allow them in their homes at a time when they did not have anywhere else to stay. After observing this, another neighbor stepped in to help by first requesting to see their medical certificates to confirm that they had tested negative for the virus. After confirming that they were Ebola-free, the neighbor invited them to live in her house until the survivor and her children were able to find a new place to live. These acts of kindness increased over time as the fear of the disease decreased and the physical health of survivors improved. Nevertheless, the semblance of normalcy this created was occasionally disrupted by the stigmatization of survivors at times when it was least expected.

Conflicts between the children of survivors and their friends sometimes led to arguments during which the latter would attempt to get an edge by making fun of the former because their parents had contracted Ebola. Used in this manner, the deployment of stigma reduced the ability of survivors and their families to respond in kind while reminding them that they were still considered to be outsiders. At the same time, it revealed the fragility of the acceptance they thought they had received as they became more removed from their experiences with the disease. Not surprisingly, these experiences reignited many of the psychological responses known to negatively affect the health of survivors.

In some ways, this summarizes what a woman in Monrovia reported she went through several months after she returned home. Before she was discharged from the ELWA hospital, she was concerned that people in her community would not be able to look past her experiences with the disease. However, she was initially relieved to discover that no one in her locality seemed to have a problem with her presence. All it took was an argument with a friend from another community for her to realize that things were not as normal as she thought. As she explained, she left the argument with a more rounded perspective of her continued vulnerability to stigma and her reaction to it:

> I was received with happiness, but only in the community where I lived. I had a friend who lived in Red Light, so when I went home, there was an argument between both of us, and she brought up the fact that I was an Ebola survivor. That word, when somebody mentions it to me, it really makes me to feel bad. It makes me feel so discouraged. So, I only tell some people or my family members that I know that I am an Ebola survivor because some of them, when you tell them you are a survivor, as soon as something small happens between you and them, they use it to insult you. Then you will start thinking about the past. So, I just do not really like to share my story with some people because when you tell them you are a survivor, they will tell you that you are lying because nobody survives from the symptoms of Ebola.

Challenging Stigma in Ebola-Affected Communities

As reports of the stigmatization of Ebola survivors spread rapidly during the second half of the epidemic, it became clear that something urgently needed to be done. Robust challenges to stigma were needed to give survivors the best chance of being socially reintegrated. However, this required action on several different fronts. Medical certificates showing that survivors had tested negative for Ebola represented only one approach used to achieve this objective. This strategy worked, but only to the extent that people were willing to accept the primacy of evidence over the reality of their own fears. In many cases, the certificates did not work as intended. Instead, they served as markers that identified people who had previously had the disease, which made them easy targets for discriminatory behaviors they would not have experienced had their status as survivors remained unknown.

Other strategies used to combat stigma started by focusing on the provision of support services and other resources. Some of these, such as counseling services, were more useful as interventions designed to mitigate the negative impacts of stigma on survivors' psychosocial well-being. Another set of strategies, including moving, discussed in the next section, was used to preempt or reduce the discriminatory reactions they received from people in their communities. Other approaches sought to directly engage the public, with the hope of promoting changes in behavior that would make communities more welcoming. Much of the work involving all these strategies was performed by NGOs with outside funding, which meant that the impacts of these interventions declined as NGO priorities changed following the end of the epidemic.

Counseling services were the most direct form of intervention used to provide services to survivors to help them cope with stigma. ETUs operated by NGOs such as Doctors Without Borders started the process even before survivors were ready to be discharged. As they prepared to return home, survivors were usually told that they should expect to be stigmatized by people who still continued to fear the disease. The process continued with volunteer counselors serving as advocates for them as they boarded the vehicles taking them home. One survivor remarked, "They will put you in the car and ask the people not to be afraid of you, and say

'This person here does not have the virus anymore. In fact, these Ebola survivors are going to be one of the main groups we will be working with to help us fight the virus.'"

After survivors returned home, NGO-run facilities were among the few places where they could seek psychosocial counseling to address the consequences of stigma. At that point, the primary focus of the counseling was to shield survivors from the negative effects of the stigma on their mental health. Without these services, stigma could have further exacerbated the emotional burdens survivors already faced, including mourning the deaths of their loved ones, coping with self-stigma, and living with other mental health complications of Ebola.

Public engagement aimed at behavioral change was used as a more macro-level strategy for combating the sources of stigma. As the first survivors began to return home and attempt to reintegrate, policymakers discovered that a major issue that needed to be confronted in anti-stigma campaigns was the spread of rumors promoting the notion that survivors were still contagious. Although the sources of rumors were difficult to identify, aid agencies devised creative methods to find them so that they could be addressed. For example, one organization in Liberia used a network of journalists and social activists to develop a "Rumor Tracker," which traced the most prevalent rumors on social media and in reports by local news organizations. These rumors were then forwarded to a hotline used by social organizers, faith-based organizations, and public officials to get a sense of the specific misinformation that needed to be debunked.[14]

Local counselors in both Liberia and Sierra Leone supplemented such efforts by making routine visits to the homes of survivors, to encourage and reassure them that the blowback they were facing was mostly temporary. This helped to shift counseling sessions away from NGO facilities to the doorsteps of survivors, where these services were most needed. Apart from providing individual-level services to survivors, the visits were also used to achieve other community-wide objectives. One of them was to continue serving as advocates by talking to people in the community to help combat misconceptions about whether survivors were still infectious.

Yemi, a young woman on the outskirts of Freetown, was one individual for whom this strategy helped as she tried to transition back into community life. The intervention was particularly needed because of the emotional turmoil and community-wide stigma she faced when she first returned home. She used to cry and feel depressed when she saw how much weight she had lost while at the ETU. Over the following weeks, Yemi noticed that neither her fellow street traders nor her former customers were coming near the stall she used to sell her wares. As she put it:

> People did not come near me. They all ran away from me. It made me cry all over again. Some of them just stayed in their shops. Others stood far away, just looking at me. I told them, "I'm alive. I did not die." But people were afraid of me. They said we had big maggots in our bodies. I told them maggots will only come out of my body after I'm dead. No maggots will climb over my body. When customers came to buy, they would throw the money towards me. When I go to buy something, the person I am buying from would ask me to drop the money down.

These reactions changed after she received a visit from a local counselor at her place of work. As she explained, "They were not coming close to me until after a counselor came to where I worked and talked to the people and told them that 'This woman no longer has Ebola.' After that, people started coming close to me, shaking my hand, and the like."

Another objective of these community visits was to combat stigma through demonstration. This demonstration involved deliberately timed physical interactions between counselors and survivors in public places that confirmed to onlookers that it was safe to touch those who had recovered. It was a strategy that not only helped to address questions about whether Ebola patients can truly recover but also to dispel the myth that locals needed to be socially distanced from survivors to avoid being infected.

Sallu, a male survivor in Freetown, provided an account that made it clear that he found the strategy to be useful. Before he was discharged, he received reports that his children and close friends back home were being stigmatized by members of his community because he had been infected. To preemptively address the problem, he asked a doctor at his ETU to accompany him home when he was discharged. This, he believed, was the proof his neighbors needed to see to believe that he had truly recovered. Although Sallu was not granted his request, a counselor living in his locality helped him accomplish the same objective. Describing the changes that followed the counselor's visit and use of demonstration, he said:

When I returned—the community had not seen anyone survive from Ebola at that time—a lot of people came out to observe what was going on when they heard that I had come home. However, they did not come near me. There was a guy there who was part of the local task force, I gave him my certificate. After he read it, he hugged me and said to my neighbors, "This guy has recovered. Do you see me hugging him? This is to show you he no longer has the disease." After that, my friends started to come near me. I did not blame them for being afraid of me.

Apart from these efforts, community leaders developed their own initiatives to respond directly to the stigmatization of survivors. These grassroots-level initiatives were among the most significant examples of how anti-stigma strategies emerged without financial assistance from outside sources. Those developing the initiatives ranged from religious clerics, teachers, work supervisors, and leaders of neighborhood organizations. For reasons that are not immediately clear, considerably more accounts of such community-led efforts to combat stigma occurred in interviews conducted in Sierra Leone than in Liberia. A possible explanation for the difference is that it was driven by the larger number of survivors in the former compared to the latter. Notwithstanding the disparity, these initiatives were very important for providing timely responses backed by locally recognized systems of leadership.

This local leadership influence was critical for addressing the stigma faced by one Ebola orphan in Freetown after he returned to school. A senior secondary school student during the epidemic, he was repeatedly bullied and ridiculed by other students after they learned that he was a survivor. In fact, the students found a creative way of labeling him to target him for stigma. Instead of referring to him by his name (e.g., John), they labelled him with a hyphenated name that combined his real name and the word Ebola (e.g., John-Ebola). He told the school principal about this when he became frustrated with how he was being treated, and the principal decided to intervene. During a subsequent school assembly, the principal decided to talk about the dangers of stigma while expressing his disapproval of the way the student was treated. Not surprisingly, the stigmatization stopped after that, allowing the student to focus on his education.

Among the most effective of these types of community-led initiatives were those developed by local chiefs. Survivors in rural areas exploited the fact that chiefs are widely seen as revered authorities who could be approached to seek redress from injustice. When chiefs addressed the problem of stigma, they did so by speaking to their subjects about the problem, which helped to change behaviors. As reported in one study, their repertoire for combating stigma was extensive. Accordingly, one chief, who had multiple survivors in his village in Sierra Leone, passed a decree that levied a fine of 500,000 Leones[15] against anyone who made fun of Ebola survivors.[16] Through local headmen, imams, and pastors, other chiefs spread messages about the need to stop the stigmatization of survivors, which was instrumental in helping survivors in their efforts to be reintegrated.[17]

Taking Matters into Their Own Hands

A final set of anti-stigma initiatives were those taken by Ebola survivors themselves. These actions were significant because they showed that survivors were not just victims depending on others to challenge the stigma they encountered. By taking action themselves, they showed that they were social actors with agency—people who took matters into their own hands to contest the everyday acts of discrimination they experienced due to the stigma of Ebola. These actions had several advantages, including the fact that they addressed stigma at the interpersonal level. Additionally, they were more immediate, occurring shortly after an instance of stigmatization. This dynamic resulted in a more immediate resolution of the problem compared to, for example, the actions taken by chiefs. Some of the actions taken by survivors were also specifically designed to prevent actual experiences of stigma.

Nondisclosure of Ebola survivor status was the most common method survivors used to achieve this objective. Many survivors had witnessed the unintended consequences of official status markers, such as medical certificates, which were intended to ease their transition into community life. Other status markers, such as identity cards issued by Ebola survivors' associations, were further supposed to unlock the benefits government officials promised in national narratives that described them as heroes and not epidemic victims.[18] However, interviews conducted in Liberia revealed that, as mentioned earlier, these identity cards were sometimes considered to be counterproductive because they merely identified survivors as targets of stigma. Similarly, some survivors in Sierra Leone believed that disclosing their status as Ebola survivors when applying for jobs, which some did to gain an advantage, had the opposite effect—making it difficult for them to get job interviews.

Nondisclosure sometimes involved being strategic in publicly associating with other Ebola survivors and, in some cases, withholding information about prior experiences with the disease while attempting to develop social relationships. For example, one survivor mentioned that she had to be discreet when attending meetings of her local Ebola survivors' group because she did not want her neighbors to know she was a survivor. Moreover, as discussed in chapter 3, the practice of nondisclosure was useful when attempting to forge romantic relationships. Notably, the practice sometimes continued after these relationships had developed into stable unions. This was strikingly apparent during an interview conducted with a male survivor in Freetown. As he talked about the problem he continued to face with stigma, he pointed to a toddler he had brought along with him and said, "You see my son over there? His mother still does not know that I am a survivor."

There was just one major problem with the strategy of nondisclosure. It was not effective in neighborhoods where community knowledge of patient histories was extensive. At the height of the epidemic, certain clues were available in communities that made it easy to distinguish between those who had the disease and those who did not. As explained by a local member of the team that conducted interviews in Monrovia, much of this had to do with the role of ambulances. As the fear of Ebola increased during the epidemic, many infected persons tried to avoid the stigma of the disease by hiding in their homes while they received care. Given the fact that ambulances were rarely used in the city before the epidemic, the only way neighbors knew someone with Ebola lived in a specific house was when their health deteriorated to the point that they had to be taken to the hospital in an ambulance. Following the departure of the ambulance, all residents of the home became targets of stigma, and they continued to be so even if those who were ill subsequently recovered from the disease.

Apart from residents, the very homes in which Ebola-infected people lived were also stigmatized. These place-based stigmas make it difficult for people connected with tainted places to hide in their communities.[19] In some cases, community residents took extreme measures to avoid such stigmatized places. In one rural community in Moyamba, Sierra Leone, where interviews were conducted, locals identified a place where someone with Ebola lived during the epidemic. It was a hut that was now stigmatized to the point that it had been abandoned. Its roof had partially collapsed, and although its main door remained open, no one went close to it. Unlike nearby huts, its yard was full of grass, which now served as a marker of the consequences of the community's fears of approaching the dwelling.

As a result of place-based stigma, many survivors chose to move to other communities where they were not well known. This strategy had several advantages. First, it increased the possibility of using nondisclosure, since the new communities were carefully selected to minimize meeting anyone survivors knew before. Second, relocation made it easier to find a place to rent, improve mental health, and conduct business in contexts with a greater likelihood of finding clients who were not afraid of interacting with survivors.

When Frances, a survivor in Liberia, talked about her experiences with stigma, it was clear that she believed her decision to relocate helped her realize many of these benefits. She still recalled how she was treated by her community when she first returned home to Monrovia. "Everyone was afraid of me," she said. "They would stand at a distance and say, 'That's the girl that had Ebola.' Even the braids I had on my head, when I asked for help to take them off, no one helped. They were afraid." Faced with the fact that her brother was the only person in the community who did not stigmatize her, she decided to move to a new neighborhood. Reflecting on how this decision changed her life, she made the following comparison between her success in avoiding stigma in her new neighborhood to the stigma she continued to face in the old one:

> For now, it has ceased because I moved. I did not tell people in the community where I moved to that I am an Ebola survivor. Where I was living before, people still stigmatize me. My female friends there, up to now, we do not talk to each other since the time after I returned from the ETU. I even called them and told them that "The people say when you come home from the ETU, when they bring you home, it is because you no longer have Ebola." However, some of them are not convinced, so I just let it be.

Relocating to a new neighborhood nevertheless came at a cost. It required developing new relationships and learning new ways of earning a living. The sustainability of new business ventures at new locations hinged on survivors' ability to develop a new client base and form new business partnerships. Furthermore, because neighborhood relocations are involuntary, they sometimes involved leaving a community where survivors owned resources such as land and moving to areas where they had none. Despite these difficulties, those who decided to leave their former communities considered these costs to be worthwhile, viewing them as much less of a problem than the stigma they would have experienced had they decided to remain in their previous communities.

Not every survivor was able to use relocation as a strategy for escaping stigma. However, some who stayed still took direct actions to challenge stigma within their own localities. In part, these actions either stemmed from their frustrations at being frequently targeted or were spontaneous reactions to blatant acts of prejudice. As such, the survivors who used these strategies justified their responses by framing them as steps taken after they had been pushed to their limits.

Take, for example, the account of a lady who was already frustrated with the negative reactions of her relatives toward her and her young child. When her cousin made things worse by making fun of her because was a survivor, she said, "[We] got into a fist fight because she was making fun of me by saying that I still had Ebola. When I lost my temper, I hit her with a wooden board. Even when my child—a nine-year-old—went near other people, they were moving away from him."

Another survivor, a widow who also lost her husband to Ebola, indicated that she was forced to act as her encounters with stigma increased. She had been bullied by her neighbors and lost friends who abandoned her because of their fear of the disease. Adding to her misery, she was no longer able to afford to live in the place where she had lived with her husband before he died. As a result, she moved in with her mother and lived in her house for a while. Other house residents, who were uncomfortable with her presence, later asked her to leave. However, she refused to back down. She said, "I insisted to stay at the house, I told them if they don't allow me to live there, I will burn the house down." When they realized that she was serious they relented but continued to keep her at a distance.

Other individual acts of agency reported by survivors varied in their complexity. While relocation was not always possible, it was sometimes possible to reduce the sense of isolation by inviting relatives from other places to move in with survivors. One person took legal action against a neighbor who had reportedly accused her of "dropping Ebola" around while she walked in the community. By "dropping Ebola," her neighbor was referring to the drops of water that spilled from buckets she carried while walking on the street. Following this accusation, she took legal action against the neighbor, who subsequently made a traditional visit to her home with community elders to apologize. As a result, she withdrew the case, relieved that her voice had been heard.

The Resilience of Stigma and the Social Consequences of Epidemics

There is no question that stigma now has less of an impact on the lives of Ebola survivors than it did during the epidemic. Yet, it continues to have implications for their social lives. Rather than resuming their involvement in their community's system of mutual dependency, many survivors remain socially isolated after being repeatedly ostracized and ridiculed. Many of the friendships destroyed by stigma also remain broken, while stigmatized places continue to be linked with the fear of Ebola. What's more, some survivors remain reluctant to disclose their status to avoid attracting the stigma of the disease. These actions are instructive, as they reflect the latent concern of survivors that the fear of the disease can still negatively affect their everyday interactions. In fact, leaders of Ebola survivor associations clearly acknowledged that the problem of stigma still exists. They said their members continue to encounter stigma in public spaces, during the course of routine activities, and while looking for jobs.

Although anti-stigma campaigns mounted by NGOs and government agencies played a vital role in recent declines in stigma, these declines are just a first step along the long road to recovery. Addressing the continued problems posed by stigma will require using a different set of strategies. Indeed, a change in approach is needed to address the gap created by changes in the funding priorities of NGOs that occurred following the end of the epidemic. As the stigmatization of nurses in health care contexts suggests, the stigma of Ebola is so deeply rooted in some communities that it may be resistant to strategies that focus solely on providing access to information. One reason for this is that many survivors come from social groups that were already stigmatized for their low socioeconomic status before the epidemic. As such, it may be difficult for them to shed the social labels used to identify them as sources of contamination.

It is also possible that anti-stigma advocates have underestimated the degree to which the fear of Ebola is now culturally rooted in West African communities. This was observed during recent trials conducted to test newly developed Ebola vaccines. In one such trial conducted in Liberia several years after the epidemic, researchers discovered that Ebola-free participants who volunteered to receive the vaccines were later stigmatized by members of their communities.[20] From the perspective of locals, receiving the vaccine was the same thing as being infected with the virus. Therefore, the volunteers were considered to be people who would soon become ill and die, which made them subject to the same negative responses that locals had toward survivors during the epidemic.[21]

These social realities will need to be addressed using a combination of strategies. For example, careful attention should be given to the routine one-on-one interactions that occur between survivors and their community members, thereby ensuring that anti-stigma messages are better suited to real-world situations. Harnessing the potential of community leaders for combating stigma is another strategy worth exploring. Unlike NGOs that leave after the end of epidemics and political leaders who change after election cycles, community leaders have a presence in their communities for much longer. Consequently, it is easy for them to take ownership of interventions that promise to improve the welfare of their residents. In addition, country-level variations in the influence of these leaders should be explored. For example, the apparent variations in the influence of these leaders in Sierra Leone and Liberia can be used as indispensable opportunities for learning what worked in one context that could be transferred to the other.

Because the residual stigma of Ebola continues, the provision of services that address its instrumental consequences for survivors should also be strengthened. Access to psychosocial counseling does not need to be curtailed because of shifts in funding priorities. Legal services need to be available to survivors to help them seek redress for their continued experiences of discrimination. Liberian survivors have taken a positive step in this direction by leveraging the skills of their colleagues who are now legal professionals. Similar initiatives should be supported to address other biases experienced by survivors. Together with other efforts, these measures could provide a cornerstone to challenge the sustained prevalence of stigma as a social consequence of the epidemic.

6 Livelihood Strategies and the Economic Consequences of the Epidemic

Of the many challenges Ebola creates for survivors as they return to their normal lives, few are as critical as the economic consequences of the virus. This does not discount the importance of stigma and the long-term health complications of Ebola. However, compared to these issues, the economic ramifications of the virus are especially concerning. The serious nature of these aftereffects is in part due to Ebola infections being mostly concentrated among people in low socioeconomic circumstances. Consequently, they were more exposed to the sum total of the negative consequences of the virus, which made it more difficult for them to recover. At the same time, Ebola created economic burdens that were directly linked to the standard protocols used for controlling the outbreak. A central part of these protocols is the requirement to destroy the personal belongings of people who have contracted the virus.[1] The rationale for the strategy is intuitive. After all, Ebola is easily transmitted through contact with infected bodily fluids, which could have touched their possessions. Nevertheless, this policy had far-reaching implications for the livelihoods of survivors as they attempted to return to their economic activities.

These implications included the problems the policy created for Titi after she was discharged from the 34 Military Hospital in Freetown. At the time, she lived in one of the many marginalized communities on the outskirts of the city that had been severely affected by the outbreak. After Titi returned home, she was shocked to discover that everything she owned had been destroyed by the health authorities. As she took stock of her losses, she discovered that they included her life savings. Titi was no different from many poor people in developing countries who do not use formal banking services. Consequently, she had saved the meager profits she earned from her work as a fish trader in a plastic bag hidden under her mattress. When her belongings were destroyed, so too was the plastic bag containing her savings. All this happened while she was at the hospital, so she only learned about her losses after she was discharged. When she returned home, she said, "I was told that the people who came to take me to the hospital burnt everything up. They took all my things, including my money and burnt them."

Losing these savings destroyed indispensable resources Titi had hoped to use to rebuild her life and support her family. She could no longer work as she used to because of chronic musculoskeletal problems, which were side effects of her infection with Ebola. The complications did not just affect what she used to do but also her ability to perform other physically demanding tasks. However, even if she was able to return to her job as a fish trader, her earnings would not have been sufficient to meet her new responsibilities. She was now a single parent with young children, and she lacked the resources she needed to take care of them. She had expected the government to step in to help support her family, but the support she hoped for was never received.

Circumstances like these have contributed to significant declines in the living circumstances of Ebola survivors, especially those in marginalized communities. In the resource-poor contexts of Liberia and Sierra Leone, people in these communities include fish traders, day laborers, and the unemployed, who are more vulnerable to the consequences of economic crises than members of the middle class. Unlike those in marginalized communities, members of the middle class are better integrated into systems of economic protection, such as formal banking services, various types of insurance, and salaried employment. As a result, when faced with economic disruptions caused by the destruction of their belongings, they are in a much better position to recover and return to their usual economic activities.

Evidence on the aftermath of epidemics accumulated over several decades has shown that these challenges are quite common among marginalized groups and can negatively affect their well-being.[2] However, these problems are also caused by factors that extend beyond personal losses. One such challenge is that the economic recovery of these groups occurs within societies that have themselves been negatively affected by epidemics. Such macroeconomic consequences were observed during the SARS epidemic, when Hong Kong's GDP declined by $3.5 billion and China's GDP growth fell by 3%.[3] Epidemics in Africa before 2014 were similarly followed by macroeconomic problems, such as declines in economic growth, reductions in tax revenues, and limits in the capacity of governments to support critical infrastructure.[4] These consequences generally filter into households, where their negative implications are felt most directly.

In both Liberia and Sierra Leone, the macroeconomic consequences of the Ebola epidemic were similarly daunting. Already among the world's poorest nations before 2014, their governments were faced with the task of balancing the need to respond to competing post-epidemic priorities with the reality of the limited resources they had at their disposal. More often than not, the priorities of survivors failed to receive the attention they deserved. For example, in Sierra Leone, the government prioritized making investments that promised to stimulate its declining fiscal indicators while making small investments in survivors themselves.[5] During periods of economic decline, such as those following epidemics, traditional African systems have helped to fill the gaps created by these shortfalls in investments.[6] However, in both Liberia and Sierra Leone, these systems were themselves negatively affected by the epidemic. While some of them have shown signs of recovery since the end of the epidemic, many survivors continue to face substantial hurdles in their efforts to confront the economic problems that have diminished their livelihoods.

Careful planning could have helped to secure an optimistic future for survivors. However, whatever planning was done was not sufficient for preventing them from experiencing the brunt of the struggle associated with supporting themselves. Experience from prior epidemics was not successfully used to anticipate the needs of survivors or to secure the resources required for ameliorating these challenges. The low socioeconomic status of most Ebola-affected populations had been established by the middle of 2014.[7] However, the policy approach that informed the long-term strategies used for their recovery failed to account for the obvious—that survivors are not able to fully rebound from the disruptions to their livelihoods without increased investments in their communities.

A closer look at the everyday lives of survivors is thus needed to fully understand how they have navigated these disruptions since the end of the epidemic. To start the process, it is important to acknowledge that the issues they continue to face are direct consequences of the epidemic's impact on their physical, social, and economic well-being. Policymakers had to have known that these impacts were on the horizon, since they had been observed in prior epidemics. Therefore, it is important to know what policymakers did (if anything at all) to address these consequences. Were the interventions they used to address the economic welfare of survivors adequate? Were these interventions sustainable? Additionally, what have residents of local communities done to facilitate the economic integration of survivors? Seeking answers to these questions does not imply that survivors should be viewed as victims who are dependent on the actions of others to survive. On the contrary, they are not. A careful analysis is therefore needed to identify what survivors have done to meet these needs and what their sources of resilience have been to develop a more rounded picture of how they have adapted to their new economic realities.

Disease Control, Property Destruction, and Material Hardships

Property destruction as a method of disease control plays an integral role in limiting the community spread of deadly viruses. In fact, there is a long history of societies using this specific method of disease control. Biblical accounts of the control of contagious diseases in ancient Israel indicate that the destruction of homes suspected to be contaminated, followed by the transfer of the debris to the outskirts of cities, was an essential part of this process.[8] Public health officials adopted similar practices in subsequent centuries as they added to their repertoire for dealing with epidemics. As such, during the plague outbreak in Europe in the late 1800s, the houses and personal property of the infected were burned to curb the spread of the disease.[9] Today, this strategy of destroying potential sources of contagion has been so effective that it is also used to control outbreaks of viruses among nonhuman animals and plants.[10]

Critics have nevertheless been concerned about the potential for this method of disease control to be abused. One such problematic use of the policy was observed during the South African plague epidemic that occurred in the late 1890s. Rather than focus on the groups that were most affected by the disease, public health officials used the strategy of property destruction extensively among Black South Africans, despite the fact that they had lower levels of plague mortality compared to White South Africans. Moreover, although Black South Africans experienced significant loss of resources as a result of the policy, they did not receive any compensation, which led to mass protests in their communities.[11]

Controlling the spread of Ebola creates a significant tension between the need to harness the health benefits of property destruction and the need to ensure that those negatively affected by the policy are not worse off than they were before. The practice is now part of the WHO's standard protocol for controlling the spread of Ebola, along with other measures such as the burning of medical waste and the safe handling of infected corpses. WHO documents specifically describe the protocol as follows: "The clothing, bedding, and other belongings of the [infected] individual should be burned."[12] While the directive makes sense, it raises two significant issues. First, as in some previous epidemics, it has the potential for abuse. In some cases, such as during the 1995 Ebola epidemic in Kikwit, the neighbors of Ebola patients developed their own interpretation of these guidelines by burning not only blankets, clothes, and beds but also the huts of those who were infected.[13] Second, the policy is not followed by a similarly detailed recommendation for how to mitigate the effects of these losses on the lives of people who had contracted the disease. In doing so, it fails to acknowledge the importance of housing, basic amenities, and the circumstances in which people live as social determinants of health.

When the 2014 Ebola epidemic occurred in West Africa, the destruction protocol was implemented without giving systematic attention to these limitations. The homes of Ebola patients were stripped bare and their clothing, beds, and other possessions were burned. In the process, they lost essential items such as kitchen utensils, tools, and furniture as well as various nonessential items, including personal mementos. Additional losses were also experienced by patients who were admitted to ETUs. Before they were discharged, they were required to give up the belongings they had with them, such as cellphones and books, to be destroyed. As in the 1995 Ebola outbreak in Kikwit, there were also times when the neighbors of survivors attempted to replicate the process by burning the homes of survivors.[14]

Regardless of how the loss of property occurs, the negative consequences for Ebola survivors largely remain the same. Precious assets and belongings that had been accumulated over time were simply burned or destroyed. Some of these, including basic furniture, were amassed over several years because of how expensive they were to purchase. This process may have involved first purchasing a bed after receiving a windfall of some sort, followed by a table here and a chair there in subsequent years, during fortuitous encounters with flea-market deals. When these belongings are destroyed, the process starts again, with one important difference: the economic conditions are defined by their inferior opportunities for earning an income, compared to the opportunities they had in the past.

Owing to these realities, some Liberian Ebola survivors compared the process of rebuilding their lives to their past experiences of starting over at the end of the country's civil war. Like the period immediately following the end of the war, survivors returned home to places that had nothing to offer other than bare floors. In these places Ebola survivors spent the first nights after their recovery, thankful that they were alive but worried about the future. Because they lacked the bare essentials at home, mundane tasks such as cooking, cleaning, and ironing became impossible to complete. Their old routines, which had supported their livelihoods, gave way to new routines as they lived among neighbors who were united by their fear of Ebola. As one survivor recalled, in the weeks that followed, the process of navigating these issues was arduous:

> Everything that we had got burned, so when we came home, to even get clothes to wear was hard for us. To even get a cooking pot to cook was hard for us, not to mention getting money to sustain this family. Buying food was hard for us. And there were other problems we had with people. Anything we touched, they didn't want to touch, so that was one of the major challenges we had.

Similar hardships were faced by survivors in Freetown, Sierra Leone, although the consequences of the policy of property destruction were more adverse among those who lived in the rural areas. The latter include poor, agricultural communities, where the destruction of property did not just lead to a loss of personal effects and savings but also to widespread losses of the tools and assets used to support survivors' subsistence occupations. Among small-scale fishermen, for example, this included the loss of fishing nets, which were among the things burned by health officials in their efforts to control the virus. In one case, the net burned was not even owned by the survivor who lived in the home. Instead, as he observed, "The fishing net I was using was rented. However, when they found out that I had Ebola, they took away everything in my house to be burnt. So, I thought the government was going to provide for us, but they did not." For this individual, therefore, the policy of destroying personal belongings led to the loss of personal property, the loss of a rented asset that was not replaced, and a likely increase in financial hardship created by the need to replace the net and return it to its owner.

Ebola Diagnosis as a Source of Material Hardship

While the policy of destroying personal belongings was widely implemented, it was not the only cause of survivors' economic problems. By itself, an Ebola diagnosis caused disruptions to economic activity that were over and beyond those caused by the policy. Being infected with the virus limited the participation of patients in productive economic activities. Within families, the presence of the virus further required the development of new responses, such as the reconfiguration of social networks that were critical for supporting their sources of livelihood. Survivors began to experience these influences almost immediately after their diagnoses. Additionally, they continued to be problematic after survivors recovered, which made it tough for them to return to their previous sources of livelihood.

At the first signs of infection, the stage was set for shifting survivors' attention away from work to survival. With their gradual physical incapacitation, the process continued with a cascading series of problems. Workers whose jobs did not provide sick days off for employees began to lose wages with each day they were admitted at ETUs. This was particularly true for self-employed business owners, whose admission at ETUs usually left them with no one to fill their roles. Each day of admission became a day without sales, and the negative consequences added up to substantial losses of earnings. Nowhere were these losses as pivotal as they were in rural areas, where agriculture is the main economic activity. Agricultural activities have two characteristics that made them susceptible to the consequences of the epidemic. First, they depend on manual labor. Second, they involve the production of perishable commodities.

The combined effects of these two characteristics were observed in the peculiar problems they caused Dembo as he recovered in rural Moyamba.

Unlike many residents in his community, he had received formal training in agriculture before starting to work as a farmer. Over the years, the training had paid off so well that he owned the only house in his village built with concrete blocks. When the epidemic started, however, he began to experience symptoms of Ebola while working on his farm and was subsequently admitted to an ETU. Upon his recovery, he attempted to resume his life as a farmer, but he discovered that things had changed for the worse. As he explained, "Because no one took care of my farm when I was in the hospital, some of my crops were destroyed, while wild animals ate the rest."

The financial quagmire created by these losses were almost unsolvable for Dembo. For one, his poor state of health made it impossible for him to cultivate his farm as intensely as he did before. In fact, he now worked on his farm less frequently than he did in the past because his doctor had informed him that he needed to take time to rest. Following his doctor's advice meant that he only worked on a few small plots of land a day, compared to the couple of acres he used to cover before he was ill. To make things worse, Dembo's financial predicament was now compounded by recent increases in the cost of living. At the time of his interview, things had become so difficult that he had used all his savings to meet his daily expenses.

Other rural survivors, such as Jallah, faced similar types of issues. Jallah lived in a village that was not too far from Dembo's. She used to run her own business, selling fresh groceries at a local market where villagers bought vegetables, fish, and other goods used for cooking. However, her business was temporarily suspended after she became sick with Ebola. When Jallah's health improved, she started to prepare to resume her work at the market, only to discover that she had lost everything. She said, "I thought I would return to my business and be well received, and that people who owed me money will be prepared to pay me. However, this did not happen." Instead, by the time she recovered, much of the inventory she kept in her store had become rotten. The rest had either been eaten by mice or used by roaches to build their nests. She still remembered the consequences of these developments as she explained what had happened:

> I could not sell [my goods] in the market. I threw them away. My business was destroyed. I also stopped seeing the people who used to help me. Right now, I

am not employed. So that's the area where I need some help because I do not have the means to start a business. I am not doing anything at the moment. Some days, I would go into the forest to pick up vegetables, because we plant some vegetables in the forests, which we use to help us. But now, it's the rainy season and things are not easy.

While rural survivors were more likely to have these experiences with perishable commodities, survivors in both rural and urban areas had one specific concern in common. They both faced health complications and the lingering effects of stigma, which continued to be the two ways through which their Ebola diagnosis still affected their ability to make a living.

At best, health problems only occasionally affected their ability to return to economic activities. Some conditions such as temporary vision loss, weight loss, and diarrhea generally improved over time, increasing the ability of many Ebola survivors to return to the workforce. But at worst, other health complications had more permanent negative effects on survivors' economic well-being that made a return to working untenable. Those affected by these serious complications included fishermen and farmers, whose health never returned to pre-epidemic levels and for whom the physical demands of their job made it virtually impossible to do the things they used to. As a result, they are now permanently excluded from the workforce.

When the survivors discussed these exclusions from the labor market, they usually provided specific explanations of how their health conditions affected their ability to work. The most common of these explanations were found in statements such as "I was not able to start working again because of my poor eye-sight," "I [now] usually have a lot of headaches," and "I was not healthy as I was before I got Ebola." Other survivors who had permanent vision loss, musculoskeletal conditions, or mental health issues described their current plight in terms of a mismatch between their desire to work and their ability to do so. As one of them stated, "I want to go back to the field, but my joints are giving me a hard time."

Many other survivors were still physically able to work. However, this ability usually concealed the indirect ways in which poor health affected their overall economic welfare. For example, physical exertion could cause flare-ups of symptoms that interrupted the workdays of those who could still work. In addition, when at work, minor mental health symptoms could sometimes distract workers from their job tasks in ways that were embarrassing. One example of this was found in an account given by a survivor who had occasional episodes of memory loss at work. He described them as occurring when "I would be saying something to my colleagues at work and they would ask me about it later, but I would have forgotten."

Extended periods of pain further affected economic activity by increasing the duration of absence from work. Many of these interruptions resulted in more than just a few lost hours of work per day. As one survivor put it, working long hours caused pain along his spine and on his sides: "I sometimes have to take a break. Sometimes this means that I have to be away from work for between 3 and 4 days before I recover." Another person with similar experiences reported that he experienced spells of dizziness. He then provided an apt example of how these spells made him feel. According to him, they felt like everything was "turning upside down," like a drunk person would feel after drinking cane juice, a local alcoholic beverage in Liberia made from sugarcane. At other times, survivors' ability to work can be affected by more than just one health complication. As yet another survivor recalled, "Sometimes my body tingles and sometimes I am confused, so I have to go home to rest before I can recover."

Besides those physical aftereffects, stigma also exerted a negative influence on survivors' economic recovery. This detrimental effect extended beyond the problems it created for those looking for jobs, which were discussed in the previous chapter. Another dimension of the influence of stigma was associated with job losses among people who were previously employed. All reports of stigma-related job losses among survivors interviewed for this study were made by those who were employed in low-status jobs. Unlike white-collar workers, they lacked formal channels for filing grievances at their places of work when such firings occurred. Self-employed workers in low-status jobs, though, were shielded from some of these experiences. Nevertheless, they were exposed to a similar type of vulnerability associated with the damaging effect of stigma on their ability to retain their previous clients. The loss of clients was primarily experienced by self-employed workers whose jobs either required physical interaction with others (for example, street traders) or relied on social relationships for them to be connected to new opportunities (for example, bricklayers).

Max, a self-employed construction worker in Monrovia, Liberia, was among the latter. Shortly after he recovered from Ebola, he realized that it had suddenly become more difficult to get new contracts from former clients than it had been in the past. These former clients were so filled with fear of Ebola that none of those who needed help were willing to rehire him. For someone like Max, who lacked access to a regular monthly salary, these reactions significantly affected his ability to earn a living. In fact, he was still able to recall the feelings of rejection he had at that time as he was going through the process:

> All of my clients who used to call me—and in this job that we do, people have to call you before you can do a job and get something from it—so, all those I was working for at the time, they rejected me. They didn't call me, they didn't find the time for me. So, I lost all my contacts, I lost all my jobs. There was nothing else I was doing, to even go to school was difficult—because I was thinking of going back to school since all my life, I had been working in construction. It was from my job as a construction worker that I was able to get something to eat. However, no one was calling me back nor was anyone willing to accept me.

Self-employed street traders in Freetown and Monrovia faced a related problem when the stigma of Ebola threatened the survival of their businesses. Customers who discovered that these traders were survivors declined to purchase goods from them because sales transactions involved physical contact. When sales declined, so did street traders' ability to accumulate capital for future investments. Additionally, stigma affected their ability to maintain some of the partnerships they had with other businesses, because few of their colleagues were interested in resuming these relationships. Ultimately, the negative pressure of stigma on their ability to be successful forced many survivors out of the street-trading business.

These various threats to survivors' livelihoods persisted as they continued to encounter financial challenges in their everyday experiences. They needed money to replace the clothes, kitchen utensils, and other personal belongings that had been destroyed to control the spread of the virus. Other responsibilities also required long-term access to resources. Adults who lost spouses were now the people everyone in their households looked to for their daily sustenance. To meet these expectations, they had to find ways to provide meals, pay school fees, and cover other household expenses. These expectations had to be met, despite the fact that some of the survivors still had health complications that required them to make regular visits to the hospital, which also required access to resources. By and large, the post-epidemic context in which these realities were experienced was one defined by the growing gap between the needs of survivors and their ability to finance these needs. To bridge these gaps, they capitalized on the relief brought by short-term aid, cultivated resources within their communities, and used innovative ways of finding access to new resources.

Relief Aid and Short-Term Sources of Livelihood

Several actors, including NGOs, family members, and residents of their local communities, took up the task of meeting the short-term needs of survivors. Having worked in prior humanitarian disasters, international NGOs were well prepared to deliver the first, and perhaps only, systematic attempt to restore survivors' livelihoods. At first, these efforts focused on replacing some of survivors' personal belongings that had been destroyed. Thus, across the affected countries, Ebola survivors received relief packages that included some combination of a new mattress, cooking utensils, and basic clothing. Occasionally, NGOs supplemented this aid with small cash allowances given either at one time or over a few months. For the most part, however, NGOs stopped disbursing these funds after about three to six months.

A few NGOs provided other types of assistance beyond what was included in these packages. For example, Caritas International provided medical and food assistance to survivors in Sierra Leone, while Doctors Without Borders assisted with the payment of school fees and the provision of small grants to Liberian survivors to help them restart their businesses. With the exception of Caritas International, which continued to provide aid to survivors in Sierra Leone several years after the epidemic, these efforts were generally short lived. As such, they did not produce the results needed to make survivors independent.

The failure to produce these results was not solely due to the actions taken by NGOs; it was further shaped by other factors, such as the negative social forces at play. A Liberian survivor reflected this in her account, in which she reported receiving a grant from Doctors Without Borders to help her restart her business selling groceries. Although she was able to start selling again, the business collapsed shortly thereafter, when customers refused to purchase her goods because of the stigma of Ebola.

Despite the fact that relief aid was mostly available for only a few months, it did help to shore up the well-being of survivors at the time it was provided. However, some observers regularly criticize this approach of giving short-term relief to people who lost virtually everything during a crisis, because of doubts about the contribution of emergency aid to long-term development.[15] As already noted, the problem with this short-term approach is that it misses opportunities for linking relief to development. Furthermore, it assumes that the victims of humanitarian disasters can bounce back on their own after relief funds expire. Because this assumption is rarely correct, it is important to move beyond the provision of relief during periods of recovery to the use of more sustainable strategies to improve the livelihoods of survivors.[16]

In addition, a careful assessment of the overall response to the needs of Ebola survivors reveals operational lapses that accompanied the process. For starters, survivors had uneven access to the aid they were supposed to receive. Two dimensions of this unevenness stand out. While survivors living in the same country had unequal access to aid, Liberian survivors and their counterparts in Sierra Leone experienced inconsistent access to specific sources of aid.

Variations in access to aid among survivors in the same country were evident among survivors in both countries. In Liberia, most survivors acknowledged receiving short-term assistance from one or two NGOs. But while some received a standard package of mattresses, bags of rice, and some perishable cooking products, others received far less or nothing at all. Listening to survivors describe what was going on at the time made it possible to identify a possible explanation for the problem. Survivors with privileged access to social networks within the NGO community received far more assistance than those without these connections.

Momoh was among the former, and he had no qualms as he boasted about how much aid he eventually received. A local leader of Ebola survivors in a low-income community near Monrovia, Momoh appeared to be known by everyone in the area. As a result of his social standing, he is usually viewed as one of the first points of contact for anyone interested in working with survivors in his neighborhood.[17] Because of his social connections, Momoh received relief from many more humanitarian organizations compared to most survivors in his community, and he proudly explained how he was able to amass these resources from NGOs as he was recovering from Ebola:

> When I came home, the first people who gave me money were from Red Cross. They gave me $50.00. The next was Special Emergency Activity to Restore Children's Hope (SEARCH). After SEARCH, Save the Children. Later, I received help from World Food Program (WFP). After, WFP, Equip Liberia. Some of them gave me food. But Save the Children gave me money, SEARCH gave me money, and Red Cross gave me money.

Survivors in Sierra Leone also reported within-country variations in access to relief aid, mostly associated with differences in place of residence. Some survivors received aid from NGOs while they were being discharged from ETUs around Freetown; others, though, who were admitted to ETUs on the outskirts of the city, received nothing at all. But a more pernicious inconsistency in access existed between urban residents and their counterparts in rural areas. Most of the survivors interviewed in rural villages in Moyamba indicated that they did not receive any aid. In fact, some of them were not even aware that this assistance was available. Others reported that they had heard that the government was going to assist them, but the help they had expected to receive never arrived. In one of Moyamba's villages, however, one survivor clarified that the government had indeed sent representatives to their area with limited relief supplies while the people there were being registered to receive comprehensive assistance. However, government officials failed to return with the aid they promised survivors after the registration process was completed.

It is important to note that the humanitarian aid survivors received was largely insufficient to meet all their needs. By any measure that compared what they lost when their belongings were destroyed with what they received from NGOs, the aid they ultimately received fell short of restoring their belongings. For example, some survivors received only one set of clothing, although all their clothes had been destroyed.[18] Similarly, the sole mattress offered to survivors was rarely enough to replace all the beds they lost in their families. As one survivor observed with disappointment, "They burned my clothes and my bed. But when we were returning home, MSF [Doctors Without Borders] only gave us two trousers, two shirts, and some peanut butter for us to manage."

The inadequacy of this response raises the question of whether relief aid is in fact meant to replace the belongings of survivors. While this issue may be up for debate, there is no doubt that a complete restoration of their belongings is what survivors expected. However, rather than accomplishing this goal, NGOs provided them with enough relief aid only to have the basic things they needed to survive. Clearly, this strategy is problematic. The plan to meet basic needs should provide a foundation for developing long-term interventions to support the livelihoods of survivors. It should not be used to offer them temporary solutions to problems that are likely to be permanent.

A second dimension of the irregular access to aid took the form of variations in the source of short-term relief received by survivors in Liberia and their peers in Sierra Leone. Arguably the biggest differences in the administration of relief aid to survivors in both countries was the role played by the government. Survivors in Liberia generally maintained that their government officials were invisible in the process. It is not clear whether this perceived lack of visible government participation was simply due to administrative inertia in Liberia's public sector. However, Liberian survivors experienced great disappointment because of this omission.

By contrast, most accounts provided by survivors in Freetown, Sierra Leone, underscored the active role played by their government officials in the provision of humanitarian assistance. According to them, the relief aid they received came both from NGO sources and from the government's Ministry of Social Welfare. Indeed, when Sierra Leonean survivors talked about the sources of support they received, most of them identified either the government or the government and NGOs such as Caritas International, WFP, and GOAL.

This positive perception of the government in Sierra Leone was due to two strategies used by the administration in power at that time to publicly associate itself with the disbursement of aid. First, each donation made by senior government representatives and every speech given about their contributions to survivors was done to attract maximum press coverage. For one survivor, therefore, it was specifically "President Ernest Koroma's wife

[who] gave us rice, beans, oil, palm oil, and mattresses." Survivors usually followed such comments with commendations about how well the president's political party supported survivors at that time, suggesting that the apparent politicization of aid by the government had its intended effects. Second, and relatedly, the government used the strategy of disbursing humanitarian relief during mass give-away programs organized by its Ministry of Social Welfare. These public events received wide coverage from the media, thereby creating an image of the government's supposed commitment to the welfare of Ebola survivors.

Yet this more active involvement of the government of Sierra Leone did not translate into sustainable solutions to meet the economic needs of survivors. Part of this inadequacy occurred because what the government provided was not necessarily different from the aid packages offered by NGOs. Government officials did provide one-time cash payments of approximately 750,000 Leones,[19] but this was not enough to make survivors economically independent. Additionally, as was the case with aid given by NGOs, most of the relief provided by the government ended after a few months. As a result, while Sierra Leonean survivors acknowledged the actions of their public officials, many of them claimed that they fell short of what the government had promised to them. This promise reportedly had included a cash payment of $5,000 that was supposed to help deliver financial security.

Material Hardships and the Continuing Struggle to Survive

When they turned their attention to their current economic circumstances, survivors generally offered narratives that had one thing in common. Their everyday experiences continued to be defined by the widening discrepancy between their present needs and their access to economic resources. On the one hand, they needed to deal with the financial implications of losing spouses, children, and close relatives to Ebola. On the other hand, the inability of many of them to work as they did before continued to deny them access to a steady source of income.

Unfazed by this discrepancy, they to continued work toward meeting their new responsibilities under tough economic circumstances. Many survivors who were now raising orphans were people living in poverty, and they were raising children who had lost parents who themselves had lived in poverty. Yet these survivors had found ways to strategically reallocate resources to ensure that none of these children went to bed hungry. In some cases, this involved making difficult choices. One example of this was the case of a survivor in Liberia, who was now taking care of the children of his deceased sister. With limited access to funds to take care of himself and his household, he could not afford the additional expense of paying for the children's education. As a result, he reallocated his resources by letting all of them drop out of school to help him meet his new obligations.

This lack of access to resources had implications that filtered into other life domains. Abandoned wives living without the support of their husbands now found it difficult to maintain the lifestyles they had before the epidemic. Many survivors were now experiencing new anxieties at the end of the month as they attempted to figure out how pay their rent. Others had forgone the few luxuries they had had before the epidemic, such a buying new dresses for Christmas or new outfits for Ramadan. These luxuries were no longer important, given their more urgent expenses.

Other economic disruptions produced somewhat unexpected consequences. For one survivor in Monrovia, these consequences originated with her landlord's decision to evict her after she was discharged, because she could not afford her rent. At the time of the interview, she lived in a squatter settlement near a large swamp in Monrovia's Montserrado County. Houses in these communities are small shacks with walls built with rusty iron sheets, held together by a few nails. The roofs are made with similar materials and are held in place with rocks to prevent them from being blown away by the wind. A major result of living in these houses, the survivor explained, was increased exposure to flooding during the rainy season. When it flooded, the banks of the swamp overflowed, which usually caused her shack to collapse. She then sought temporary accommodation from neighbors whose shacks were still standing, which made it easier for her to rebuild her shack.

Other challenges surfaced as well. With high unemployment in Liberia and Sierra Leone, even survivors who were able to work to find had difficulty securing jobs. With the departure of the few NGOs that had provided start-up grants for businesses, few alternative sources of business capital existed other than banks, but most survivors in poor communities did not have the collateral needed to qualify for loans. The few survivors who did have such collateral needed to take additional steps to success-fully invest the money they received. Accordingly, setting up businesses required them to be available for work, have a product that was in demand, and take advantage of other factors that were beyond their control. For some, these other factors included being able to run their businesses despite their poor health. As one survivor in Liberia recalled:

> Even this shop I have now was because of credit I was able to get from the bank. There was nobody else to help me. [But] we are still suffering; some of us are still dealing with different illnesses. For me, it's my eyes. I can't see well. And my heart beats fast, so there is no way I can turn around to help myself with this.

Living in a rural area created an additional set of burdens. Some farmers who walked away from agriculture when they were infected found it difficult to return because the lack of capital made it impossible to successfully cultivate crops again. To explain why capital was important, one farmer said, "What makes farming work is money. You have to buy seeds and pay people to prepare the land for you." Apart from this, capital was also needed to buy fertilizers and to sustain the families of farmers until the harvest was ready. In most cases, the latter is achieved using food reserves from the last year's harvest, which provide sustenance until the end of the growing season. For this system to work, however, the reserves need to be restocked every year, which is something that survivors who had been away from farming for a long time had not been able to do.

Rural areas also had fishermen who were either no longer employed or were not as productive as they were before. This hardship was not always due to their inability to replace their destroyed fishing nets. New health conditions, such as the loss of vision and increased sensitivity to low temperatures, made it difficult for them to work in the open waters. Unlike big cities like Freetown and Monrovia, where some alternatives to manual labor exist, rural areas have fewer alternatives for survivors with these health problems.

Making Ends Meet in the Years After Recovery

Confronting these challenges has required survivors to adapt to their circumstances by developing new strategies to continue with their lives.

They have done so by leveraging community resources when available, increasing their resourcefulness when possible, and exploring new ways to make ends meet. This process has evolved over several years since the end of the epidemic. In the early part of this period, family members who were not deterred by stigma offered the most important source of community resources. They provided small cash gifts, food, and other kinds of supplies as a way of helping survivors transition back into their community. As a result, some survivors reframed their perspective on who they considered to be true members of their families. Survivors took extreme care to differentiate between those they considered to be real family members—that is, those who provided for them during hard times—and those who, by their inaction, failed in their time of need.

Neighbors supported survivors less frequently than families did. Occasionally, relatively affluent neighbors supported survivors in more substantial ways. Some of these neighbors were not only distinguished by their wealth but also by the fact that they showed up at a time when many people had misgivings about interacting with survivors. A young man in Monrovia's Sector 2 reported one such interaction, where a local leader helped his family after they returned home from the ELWA hospital:

> A local philanthropist came and assisted us with some food before we started living a better life. He was the first person who gave his support. He was the representative of district 17, Mr. William Darket. He gave us 2 bags of rice and some cash. That's what we started to hang on to before the NGOs started coming.

Over time, relatives and community benefactors provided less support as NGOs increased their involvement in the provision of aid. With the subsequent departure of NGOs, however, support from both groups changed in very different ways. For the most part, a few relatives continued to provide support to survivors, but mainly to those who had little means to support themselves. Within communities, economic support for survivors has largely disappeared, especially from neighbors who witnessed the disbursement of relief aid. When neighbors learned what was in these aid packages, they perceived that survivors were now wealthy. Consequently, some neighbors argued that it was time to reverse the direction of support and for survivors to share their newfound wealth with them. While these neighbors misperceived the survivors' economic status, the error was pervasive enough to create tense relationships with the people survivors continued to approach for economic assistance.

Compared to Liberia, the false perception that survivors had amassed wealth was more prevalent in Sierra Leone, where the government actively publicized the aid it gave to survivors. To be sure, the one-time payment of about 700,000 Leones that survivors received was relatively small to support a middle-class family; however, it was a substantial amount for residents of poor communities. Within these contexts, Ethel, a young female survivor, described some of the consequences of this perception of wealth. As she stated, "Some people think we have a lot of money because of the help we received after we recovered. This is [also] a problem for some of us, even when we go out looking for jobs. However, we don't have money. Even when you have a boyfriend, he does not trust you because he thinks you have money but are hiding it from him." Ethel went on to discuss another reason why the perception that she was rich was flawed. After receiving the one-time payment of around 700,000 Leones, she decided to start her own business to give herself a more reliable source of income. However, the business collapsed after thieves stole her goods, which left her unemployed and without the ability to provide for her family.

Since community members, government agencies, and NGOs backed out of the business of providing relief, the struggle to make ends meet has become an enduring feature of the lives of survivors. Those without white-collar jobs have had to explore new ways of addressing their financial problems. Some of the best strategies used to achieve this goal have involved demonstrations of survivors' creativity and sense of agency. Additionally, these strategies have underscored survivors' determination to circumvent the effects of stigma while gleaning resources from a patchwork of methods to meet their needs.

Circumventing the economic consequences of stigma involved the use of strategies that were simply extensions of those used to avoid stigma. For example, street traders used the flexibility they have in determining where they conduct their business to stop selling their wares in neighborhoods where people knew who they were. Instead, those street traders moved to other neighborhoods, where no one knew about their history with Ebola. Additionally, after realizing that disclosing their Ebola survivor status when applying for jobs had a negative effect on their chances of employment, many survivors embraced the strategy of nondisclosure to increase their likelihood of being called for interviews.

Most survivors, however, previously worked outside the formal labor market. For them, the road to economic progress involves doing various things, such as performing an occasional odd job for a neighbor, working as a day laborer, or joining the army of street traders in Freetown or Monrovia, selling everything from a pack of gum and used clothes to boiled eggs and fried fish. While the similarities between the activities in these cities are important, differences also exist in the methods survivors use to earn an income.

For example, survivors in Freetown frequently talked about their efforts to leverage the meager resources they earn from their small economic ventures to obtain the larger payouts offered to participants in the micro-credit practice of *osusu*. In general, osusu groups are formed with small circles of trusted friends, coworkers, or neighbors who contribute as little as the equivalent of $5 to a common pool at frequent intervals (e.g., each month). Group members (for example, five people) then take turns to collect the total purse (in this case, $25) at the end of each period, which sequentially gives each person access to a larger sum of money that could be used to make bigger purchases. Community members have long used osusu groups, which go by several additional names,[20] as a strategy for poverty alleviation across Africa. As such, it is not surprising that they now play a critical role in helping survivors access funds to invest in their own development.

Musa, who was orphaned at age 17, combined funds raised from one such group as well as other sources to accumulate money to pay for his education. After losing 11 family members to Ebola, he struggled to finish his final year in secondary school, which was also the first time he was living without his parents' support. Realizing the challenges that lay ahead, Musa began to fend for himself, first by working as a day laborer in a local market in the east of Freetown. From the earnings he received from his job, he paid the fees required for him to take the West African Senior School Certificate Examination, which he needed to pass to graduate from secondary school. After that, he used earnings from a second job, as a street trader, to make osusu contributions. When it was his turn to collect money from the osusu pool, he used these resources to fund his application to college. The overall process was meticulously executed, and Musa proudly described it to show how fortunate he was to beat the odds:

> I no longer had someone to pay for me. And the year I was discharged was the year I was promoted to Senior Secondary School level 3. I was all by myself hustling. I would go to Dove-Court market and work as a day laborer. When people needed someone to carry heavy loads, I would do it for them and they would pay me 2 or 3 thousand Leones. I saved this money. I used to it to buy a private WASSCE form. I studied hard and took the exam. When the results came out, I got the requirements that I needed. At that time, I also had another business I was doing, and I participated in an osusu group. The requirement was to deposit 50k Leones every day. So, when I gathered my earnings from the group, it came to almost 5 million Leones. So, I used these funds to purchase an application form for the University of Sierra Leone. I applied and was accepted. So, that what I used the funds for.

Similarly, Dana, another survivor in Freetown, used her participation in an osusu group as one of several methods to navigate a common problem that survivors faced after they were discharged. After she returned home from the hospital, she found out that she did not have any funds to pay her rent. Although her landlord was not among those who stigmatized their tenants, he insisted that rent must be paid, regardless of whether Dana was a survivor. She said,

> I did not have money to pay rent, so my landlord laughed at me. He said that was not his problem. I found things very difficult. Every day, he was on me for his rent. That's why I took my good clothes to town and sold them. I also sold the bag of rice I had to raise the money. I also became more serious about my business selling cold water, blocks of ice, and the like. And I participated in osusu. When it was my turn to receive money from the pool, I made sure that I took out his rent first.

None of the Liberian survivors interviewed reported that they participated in similar groups. However, they had a specific livelihood strategy that they used far more frequently than their counterparts in Sierra Leone. Specifically, they participated widely in various aspects of the new health-related enterprises that emerged from the epidemic. Two such enterprises were the provision of health care to survivors and paid Ebola-related research.

Much of this work on the provision of health care for survivors started during the epidemic. Back then, NGOs setting up ETUs were quick to employ evidence from prior epidemics showing that people who had recovered from the virus were immune to the disease and could thus be employed to do basic tasks to support infected patients. The practice was generally used in Guinea, Liberia, and Sierra Leone. And although these opportunities disappeared after the end of the epidemic, they laid the foundation for expanding survivors' participation in the broader Ebola research enterprise.

PREVAIL in Liberia provides the best example of how this expansion of research fostered the continued involvement of survivors in funded Ebola studies. Early in its operations, the organization employed a small number of survivors, providing them with a source of income. However, the financial nexus of its relationship with survivors was most appropriately found in the cash incentives it offered to those enrolled in its studies. Survivors described a typical research subject's visit to PREVAIL's offices as requiring them to go through several tests, after which they received approximately $30 for showing up as well as reimbursement to cover their transportation costs. Other researchers conducting health-related studies with Ebola survivors also provided cash incentives. However, none of these studies have lasted as long as those conducted by PREVAIL.

Accumulating cash incentives by participating in multiple studies provided survivors with a modest source of income. However, they realized that this dependence on incentives was not a sustainable strategy for improving their livelihoods. For one, it was correctly seen as the product of a broken system—one that had no strategy for continuing to provide care for survivors and that had done nothing to assist them in becoming economically independent. Continuing to use incentives further risked turning them into professional research subjects, who kept looking forward to the next study that offered cash benefits. Some Liberian survivors expressed an even more salient concern about these studies. They saw the cash incentives offered to them as distractions that attempted to shift their focus away from the fact that none of these studies had provided long-term solutions to their economic problems.[21] Arguably the best expression of these frustrations was offered by a survivor who said:

> They are always taking statements from us; in the end, they use them for their own purposes. However, we really need support; when they come they shouldn't go to any leadership [of Ebola survivors' associations]. We don't need [their] leadership, because when you go to our leaders we don't hear anything [after that]. This is not the first, second, third, fourth nor the fifth study we have participated in. However, we really need help, survivors really need help. When we see our colleagues [languishing] in the streets, that really gets to us because we need help. During these past five years, we have not realized anything positive [from these studies]; they will only come and talk. Then, they give us a half bag of rice, five dollars, or something else, and go.

One only needs to consider the current plight of marginalized Ebola survivors to understand the basis for these frustrations. These survivors include people who have accumulated debts in their efforts to replace the things they lost when their belongings were destroyed. They include the many survivors who now live as homeless beggars on the streets of Freetown and Monrovia. In rural Sierra Leone, they include people who can no longer work and, as a result, have encouraged family members to migrate to Freetown, where they could look for work and send their earnings back home. As survivors talked about their peers who had died in poverty, had experienced severe mental health issues, or had turned to illegal activities to support themselves, it became clear that their frustrations are deeply rooted. Yet, much of this frustration could have been avoided with a comprehensive strategy to help survivors develop their ability to support themselves.

Sustainable Livelihoods for Survivors of the Ebola Crisis

Equipping survivors to meet their basic needs is a practical matter that that lies at the heart of the task of reintegrating them into their communities. At worst, such measures would ensure some form of continuity in their socioeconomic circumstances; that is, survivors would be able to continue living their lives where they left off and maintain the economic strategies they had before the start of the epidemic. At best, interventions that address their livelihoods should provide a useful foundation for improving their economic circumstances. When correctly executed, such interventions can improve overall well-being in the places where survivors live as well as tackle the structural problems that made them vulnerable to the consequences of the epidemic in the first place.

So far, neither of these objectives has been achieved. On the contrary, the well-being of many survivors has declined. Those in the lowest strata of society before the crisis have become dislocated from their usual sources of economic activity. In the process, the resources they had cultivated for adapting to their marginalization have largely been lost. At the same time, their economic dislocation can be seen as surprising, given what was already known about the consequences of Ebola infection from prior epidemics. The old but successful strategies used to respond to these outbreaks have not been finely tuned to provide more robust interventions to improve the lives of survivors. We need new strategies to ensure that future interventions into epidemics are not limited to the provision of relief aid to survivors after they return home from hospitals. That way, survivors would at least be able to return to the level of well-being they lived with before their health crises.

Providing care for the many patients who recovered from the virus was arguably one of the most significant accomplishments observed during the 2014 West African Ebola epidemic. Without the investments needed to make these survivors economically independent, however, they are likely to resort to using survival strategies that will increase their risk of interacting with disease vectors that could fuel the next epidemic. For this reason, it is vital for policymakers to strengthen the vulnerable communities where survivors continue to live. What we see from the accounts of Ebola survivors, however, is that many of their communities are far from this future ideal. On the contrary, these communities have become contexts where survivors experience a decline in living standards. Sadly, the only improvements in living standards that occurred during this epidemic were those linked with misuse of donor funds by officials in relief organizations.[22]

Meanwhile, a few signs of hope exist. Many survivors have shown a remarkable ability to navigate through tough economic conditions. Some have been able to bypass the negative effects of stigma on their ability to work effectively. Others have adapted their work patterns to reconcile their physical limitations with the labor demands of their occupations. Still others have taken advantage of existing systems of subsistence more systematically than they did in the past. As a result, they have been able to leverage their sparse resources in ways that have allowed them to do more with less. While their use of these strategies is commendable, it is important to note that these options are not available to all survivors. However, by harnessing the potential of the opportunities that are available, survivors have shown a significant degree of success living without the help of NGOs. It is important to build on these efforts to improve their lives even further. Without ongoing efforts, the economic crises experienced by those the disease affected most will continue.

7 Beyond Medical Responses

When first responders arrived on the scene just after the first plane crashed into the World Trade Center's North Tower on September 11, 2001, little did they know that this was the start of a series of terrorist attacks on US soil. By the time the attacks were over, hundreds of first responders had arrived at various scenes of destruction found across three states. Along with volunteers, they rescued the injured, helped to keep the peace, and recovered the remains of those who had died from these devastating events. They continued to do so for several weeks after the attacks had ended. During this period, they were exposed to carcinogenic airborne pollutants such as toxic dust particles, smoke, and fumes.[1] The effects of these pollutants were extensive but were primarily observed in New York City, where they affected the lives of first responders and residents. The final tally of victims included approximately 2,977 people who died as a direct result of the September 11 attacks.[2] Added to this are more than 18,000 people afflicted with various chronic conditions. Among the sick were people who developed cardiovascular disease, cancer, gastroesophageal reflux, and mental health conditions such as post-traumatic stress disorder and suicidal ideation.[3]

Compared to the medical consequences of the September 11 attacks, the social consequences received very limited media coverage, although they were equally important. First responders had disabilities that required them to develop new ways of navigating social spaces. Families affected by the attacks included those that were reconfigured as a result of the death of parents, siblings, and spouses. Along with these deaths was the loss of income from breadwinners who had lost their lives. Furthermore, the chronic health problems of many victims negatively affected their incomes due to their inability to return to the jobs they had before.

While the response of the US government to these issues was imperfect, it provided a valuable template for bridging the gap between the medical and social responses to humanitarian disasters. At the core of this response was the establishment of victims compensation mechanisms that addressed two major objectives. The first Victims Compensation Fund, established in 2001, provided families with money that was intended to approximate the lost earnings their loved ones would have received had they not died during the attacks.[4] This gave them access to resources that were essential for bringing them closer to the living standards they had before September 11. In subsequent years, the US government expanded the compensation program to address a second objective, namely the health problems of people who had chronic conditions associated with the attacks.[5] Since then, victims who continue to live with long-term health complications have had access to new resources that could be used to get extended care from medical facilities.

At the start of the COVID-19 pandemic, it was easy to revisit this dual approach to respond to its consequences and plan for long-term interventions to help those most affected. One of the first US government responses was to provide various types of resources to bring relief to Americans whose economic well-being had been negatively affected. These resources came in the form of interventions such as economic impact payments, rent relief, and economic assistance to businesses.[6] In addition, the US government made what was arguably its most important response to the medical consequences of the pandemic by providing billions of dollars to support the development and distribution of COVID-19 vaccines. In general, this two-pronged approach was in line with the strategies used by other Western countries to address the consequences of the pandemic.

Toward the end of the pandemic, the US government attempted to develop a more institutionalized response to the impacts of COVID-19 compared to those provided just after it started. During the first session of the 117th US Congress, Representative Adriano Espaillat introduced the COVID-19 Victims Compensation Fund Act, which proposed to develop a mechanism for addressing the losses linked to the "harms resulting from suffering from COVID-19."[7] The act defined losses as monetary and non-economic losses that included, among other things, physical pain, mental anguish, loss of companionship, and injury to reputation. This definition was broad enough to cover many long-term health and social problems usually observed in the aftermath of epidemics. Although the act was not passed into law, it represented an acknowledgement of a simple reality— the need to address the social welfare of those affected by epidemics continues even after these events are over. Moreover, the act reinforced the significance of using a two-pronged strategy that addresses both the medical and social needs of the victims of epidemics.

Justifications for the Two-Pronged Approach

At first glance, it is easy to dismiss these responses to humanitarian crises because of their high associated costs. For example, the US government spent more than $7 billion to care for the victims of the 9/11 terrorist attacks.[8] Additionally, it spent more than $1 trillion to address the various consequences of the COVID-19 pandemic. Liberia and Sierra Leone do not have resources of this magnitude. However, this should not distract us from the merits of the dual strategy since there is no substitute for addressing both the medical and social consequences of epidemics.

While reasons abound for adopting a similar approach to respond to epidemics in developing countries, three of these are among the most important and constitute the core of the main arguments made in this book. First, regardless of where epidemics occur, they most often have long-term negative consequences for the lives of those affected. This was as true of victims affected by historical epidemics such as the Plague of Athens as it is for Ebola survivors and survivors of the COVID-19 pandemic. Given these long-term consequences, most approaches that use specific dates and formal announcements to mark the end of epidemics are misleading. Although they are important to mark the end of the phase of rapid rates of disease transmission, their focus on specific endpoints ignores the fact that epidemics continue to affect lives long after they are declared to be over. When these long-term consequences are ignored, it is easy to give more attention to medical responses than social responses, because of the significance of the former for stopping the spread of disease.

A better way of understanding these dynamics is to consider the consequences of epidemics as extending through various phases. Some have used a similar approach that distinguishes among phases of epidemics associated with changes in the number of infections.[9] The main advantage of understanding the consequences of epidemics as occurring in phases is that it acknowledges the reality that those who recover from infections continue to experience important transformations in their social lives even after epidemics have ended.

A second justification for the two-pronged approach is that, compared to existing approaches, it is better suited for recognizing the fact that the negative effects of epidemics are usually concentrated among socially marginalized populations. As already noted, a similar concentration of the consequences of COVID-19 was observed among racially marginalized groups in the West. However, when epidemics occur in developing countries, their consequences for the socially marginalized take on an added level of significance. The main reason for this is that marginalized groups in developing contexts live in countries that are themselves marginalized from the global economic system. Moreover, as observed during the Ebola epidemic, many marginalized groups in African countries live in extreme poverty. When confronted with the brutal results of epidemics, they fall into deeper levels of poverty than before, in contexts without the same level of resources for protecting their well-being as those found in Western societies.

Additionally, the two-pronged approach is justified because of its potential for using the assets of survivors to develop comprehensive responses to the social consequences of epidemics. The fact that most Ebola survivors are poor and powerless does not mean that they have nothing to contribute to addressing these consequences. On the contrary, the accounts described in earlier chapters show the various things they have already begun to do to make these contributions. Current approaches for addressing these issues usually discount the contributions of survivors in favor of the contributions of humanitarian organizations. However, the latter typically use top-down strategies that are best for deploying technologies suited for addressing the medical consequences of epidemics. By contrast, the use of dual intervention strategies that harness the contributions of survivors can shift attention from top-down approaches to new strategies appropriate for local communities.

Achieving these ideals will require more than just developing new policies. Policy development must be accompanied by the provision of resources over a period of time that matches the duration of the needs found among the most affected victims. More than two decades after the end of the September 11 attacks, for example, those affected by these events continue to have access to the resources provided by the US government to address their needs. Similarly, most epidemics have victims whose lives are disrupted in ways that make it impossible for them to resume their lives in the short term. As such, while long-term commitments of abundant resources are ideal, the disruptions faced by victims are too extensive to wait for the ideal resources to be available; governments should start with the resources that already exist.

Clearly, contemporary responses to epidemics need to be expanded beyond the primary goal of addressing medical outcomes. However, most international responses to global epidemics rarely extend beyond this aim. There is no evidence that the two-pronged strategy was used to develop responses to the epidemics of the Zika virus, SARS, or the Sudan virus disease. Instead, the default approach used for these emergencies was to use conventional strategies that pay scant attention to how epidemics affect other dimensions of human life. The problem is particularly worse in developing countries where outbreaks of diseases such as tuberculosis, Lassa fever, and Ebola are usually addressed with clinical interventions, with little regard for the social consequences for people living in poverty.

Sadly, therefore, it is in countries where epidemics can cause the most negative social disruptions that the emphasis on improving the circumstances of the poor is lacking. This limitation can lead to disparate patterns of recovery between regions during global epidemics. The best example of this was observed during the 2014 Ebola epidemic. Africans who were infected by the virus faced more obstacles to recovery than their Western counterparts during this period. A typical survivor in Liberia, for example, had less access to the resources needed to support their recovery compared to Amber Vinson and Nina Pham, two of the multiple Americans who were infected with Ebola during the crisis.[10] Moreover, health complications of the virus are more consequential in Africa, where agriculture, which requires high levels of manual labor, is the predominant economic activity, compared to the United States, where the service sector predominates.

When modest attention is given to addressing social issues in developing countries, survivors are faced with no choice but to employ survival strategies known to increase the risks of new epidemics. For example, survivors may forage in forests more extensively, use polluted water sources more frequently, and engage in similar activities that destroy the resources in their communities. The longer these issues are ignored, the more difficult it will become to develop an environment that protects population health in developing countries.

Policy attention should thus be given to providing local communities with the resources they need to develop the basic systems required to support social recovery. To some extent, the process has already begun. In 2020 the African Development Bank, through its Post Ebola Social Investment Fund, provided funds to the government of Sierra Leone to increase investment in the development of community workers, social protection workers, and people with disabilities in Ebola-affected communities.[11] Similar funds were provided to the governments of Liberia and Guinea to help them restore social services and revive local economic opportunities in their Ebola-affected communities. However, such investments tend to be the exception rather than the rule. New interventions are thus needed to make such resources available to other countries to assist them in rebuilding the social infrastructure of their communities as they recover from epidemics.

African Contexts and the Peculiarities of Ebola Survivors

Notwithstanding the insights provided by the Western response to the COVID-19 pandemic, the parallels between the pandemic and the Ebola epidemic only go so far. For starters, it is impossible to ignore the huge difference in economic development found between the countries where they occurred. The robust economies of the West provide a stronger foundation for recovering from the macroeconomic consequences of these crises compared to the economies of West Africa. Without a strong macroeconomic foundation, survivors in developing countries will continue to find it difficult to sustain themselves in contexts with labor markets that provide few alternatives for those who are unemployed.

Additionally, COVID-19 survivors in the West have access to far more modern institutions and effective systems of social protection compared to Ebola survivors in West Africa. For example, legal institutions in the

West provide clear avenues for seeking redress from the injustices caused by stigma. Western financial institutions furnish business owners with access to critical services needed for resuming their disrupted operations. Because Western health institutions are well developed, they can offer a minimum threshold of services for survivors living with complications of COVID-19 that exceed the threshold available to Ebola survivors in West Africa.

These differences are important for two reasons. First, they show that resilient institutions are needed to accelerate the process of social recovery. Even though many Western institutions were affected by the COVID-19 pandemic, they recovered relatively quickly and can now provide services for survivors to help them do the same. The same cannot be said of modern institutions in Liberia and Sierra Leone, as many of them were barely functional before the start of the Ebola epidemic. Second, the differences suggest that even if Western governments had not provided new funds to meet the needs of victims of the pandemic, their citizens would have had access to other options that would have helped them recover from its consequences. Many US social security systems provide survivor benefits to the children and spouses of people who are deceased. Furthermore, unemployment benefits are available to most Western citizens who lose their jobs.

These services are largely unavailable to survivors in Liberia and Sierra Leone. For example, practically no unemployment benefits are available to citizens of these countries who become unemployed. Furthermore, as currently constituted, their social support systems have serious limitations. One of them is that their institutions are relatively new. Liberia's current social insurance program was developed in 2017, around the end of the Ebola epidemic, and has not yet implemented a system to start payments for some benefits.[12] Another limitation is that these systems tend to be exclusionary. Sierra Leone's system, which is also relatively new, mostly excludes workers in the informal sector, where most Ebola survivors were employed before the epidemic.[13] Additionally, in Liberia, eligibility for disability benefits requires payment into the system for at least 60 months (5 years) before the disability began. This requirement effectively excludes many survivors with disabilities, as they would not have paid into the system before the start of the Ebola epidemic unless they could afford the payments.

African Ebola survivors appear to be further distinguished by their experiences with the long-term health complications of the disease. In some ways, this is similar to the experiences of survivors living with the symptoms of Long COVID. However, while the consequences of Long COVID have not been studied extensively, there are several reasons to believe that the health complications of Ebola survivors could involve more challenging experiences.

For example, the medical complications associated with Ebola infections are particularly debilitating, ranging from blindness and musculoskeletal conditions to neurological ailments and reproductive health issues. Moreover, there is no question that the daily experiences of dealing with health problems in Africa are more onerous than dealing with them in the United States, given the general lack of access to care in the former. A decade after the end of the Ebola epidemic, we also know that the health complications of Ebola do indeed last for multiple years. At this point, it is not known whether people who suffer from Long COVID will continue to experiences these challenges over the next decade.

Additionally, Ebola survivors and survivors of the COVID-19 pandemic differ in their experiences with stigma. In fact, one can argue that the role of stigma in shaping the experiences of Ebola survivors is among the most pernicious social consequences of epidemics observed in recent years. This is not to say that the experiences with stigma observed during the COVID-19 pandemic were insignificant. However, compared to the experiences observed during the pandemic, which mainly targeted groups presumed to be responsible for the spread of the disease, the stigma of Ebola directly affects persons who were infected with the virus themselves. With the exception of the experiences observed during the HIV/AIDS crisis, there is arguably no systematic evidence showing that the stigma observed during recent epidemics affects survivors in subsequent years to the extent that it continues to do among Ebola survivors in West Africa.

Owing to the problematic messages about the dangers of Ebola used in disease prevention campaigns, the stigma of the disease is still used to target former patients in ways that exclude them from society. The fear of Ebola is so serious that it is now incorporated into local understandings of the relationship between infection and death. However, communities in West Africa are not alone in their fear of the disease. The social understanding of Ebola and its association with death extends to other parts of the world, where it is still found in popular narratives that promote its relationship with physical contamination.[14] Yet, these problems are not insurmountable. Past experiences of dealing with the stigma of HIV/AIDS show that stigma can be mitigated by interventions that can help to change perspectives of disease over time.

Finally, Ebola, along with many other infectious diseases in developing countries, do not receive the attention they deserve from the institutions that have the power to make the most positive difference during epidemics. This limitation has substantial consequences. As a result of the large amount of resources committed to tackling the spread of COVID-19 during the pandemic, a vaccine for the disease was developed within one year after the start of the outbreak. On the contrary, even though the first Ebola outbreak occurred around 1976, it took more than 40 years for a vaccine for the disease to be developed. This disparate attention given to these viral diseases may partly account for the lack of attention given to the social effects of epidemics in developing countries. However, all is not lost. Policymakers should continue to encourage progress toward finding solutions to the challenges posed by infectious diseases in these countries, since doing so will foster the development of appropriate interventions for improving global health.

Elevating Social Issues in Policy Interventions

Making social issues a priority for policy intervention will require global humanitarian organizations to adjust their ways of doing business. This should start by developing robust links between short-term and long-term interventions. At best, NGOs should reframe the distinction between the two to give them the same level of attention. Slight adjustments may, however, be required in developing countries to provide more attention to the latter than the former. In these countries, the social disruptions caused by epidemics can be so extensive as to make an equal emphasis on both types of interventions impractical. At worst, public health institutions should take gradual steps to elevate social issues in the planning and implementation of policy. This goal can be achieved by providing similar kinds of resources for both types of interventions to prevent donors from focusing too highly on medical interventions when the signs of an epidemic appear.

Building connections between both types of interventions should be done seamlessly to eliminate unnecessary interruptions in the provision of essential services. Survivors who have been discharged but continue to experience health complications should be automatically enrolled in programs that begin to give them access to long-term care. Strong connections between short-term and long-term policies would also address survivors' concerns about interruptions in their access to counseling services after epidemics are over. Similar connections could be used to ensure that job training programs are available to facilitate their transition to service-related occupations when diminished health prevents their return to manual jobs.

Some of these connections were developed after the end of the Ebola epidemic but were not allowed to extend over a long period of time. Similarly, problems with program development negatively affected survivors' transition to their communities. For example, many of those who participated in job training programs were trained for jobs such as soap-making and gara-dying that already saturate local labor markets. The social impacts of these programs can be increased by expanding the range of occupations survivors are trained for to increase their competitiveness in the job market. Ultimately, the goal of such programs should be to make survivors productive enough to increase their contributions to development. But this can only be achieved if they are trained to become truly independent and not abandoned when program funds no longer exist.

All of these policies and programs will require resource commitments that are higher than the commitments usually made to epidemics in developing countries. If we learned anything from the HIV/AIDS crisis, it is that the long-term outcomes of patients can be improved when a significantly large amount of resources are available. In 2003, the US government provided billions of dollars for the development of long-term solutions to the crisis as part of the President's Emergency Plan For AIDS Relief (PEPFAR) program. Over the past two decades, the program has provided more than $100 billion to fund HIV/AIDS programs, saving thousands of lives.[15] The resource commitments needed to address the consequences of small-scale epidemics are unlikely to be as large as those made by the PEPFAR program. However, they should be meaningful enough to cover the extended time it would take to make a difference in the lives of survivors.

This dynamic does not mean that governments in poor countries should be excused from making commitments to help their own citizens. While they may not have similar access to large inflows of funds, they could take other practical steps that are relatively affordable. This could include using a percentage of their existing budgetary allocations to provide services to survivors. For example, in Liberia and Sierra Leone, officials could reserve some of their existing government scholarships given to college students for Ebola survivors who no longer have relatives to finance their education. A similar strategy could be used to give survivors access to health services, job opportunities, and funds for community development. When possible, advocates should encourage governments in developing countries to make new funding commitments to complement these efforts and expand the range of services they provide.

Several direct changes should be made to the public health strategies used to combat the spread of epidemics. The first is revisiting how messages used in disease prevention campaigns are developed. As observed during the Ebola epidemic, an undue emphasis on the fact that Ebola had no cure reinforced the stigma associated with the disease. Disease prevention messages should instead focus on the practical steps needed to stop the spread of disease and the treatment options available to those who are infected. Second, the existing policy on the destruction of the personal belongings of infected persons to prevent the spread of disease needs to be revised. This process can be improved by using the same level of commitment employed to enforce the policy to promote efforts to replace what was lost in the process. It may not always be possible to replace all belongings destroyed over a short period of time. However, governments and NGOs should prioritize the needs of those who were most affected by the process when resources are disbursed to help survivors recover.

Since survivors have demonstrated that they can actively participate in addressing the social problems created by epidemics, more should be done to incorporate them in the development of long-term solutions to these problems. When confronted with stigma, they confronted the backlash they experienced by acting to mitigate its consequences. Faced with a lack of resources to make investments, they turned to traditional microcredit systems to find alternative ways of accumulating resources. Even though they had limited resources of their own, some also stepped up to care for children orphaned by Ebola and other survivors who were less fortunate than themselves. Together, these experiences show the agency that survivors can employ to advance the process of social transformation when given an opportunity to do so.

Rather than use Ebola survivors to address these social issues, humanitarian institutions have traditionally appropriated their contributions to advance the medical dimensions of recovery. They have done so by approaching survivors to donate plasma used for treating other infected patients, hiring them to provide care for patients admitted to ETUs, and asking them to participate in clinical trials to study other aspects of the disease. This list of opportunities should be expanded to build on the social resources that survivors have at their disposal. NGOs and government programs can achieve this objective by integrating survivors when planning new social programs, developing community outreach activities, and identifying future program beneficiaries.

Community residents represent another set of resources that could be used to advance social recovery, partly because they are present in the contexts where these problems are experienced. The process of tapping these resources could start by leveraging the contributions of local leaders. Local chiefs, religious leaders, and politicians have a level of credibility that demands the attention of community residents during periods of crisis. This explains why they were so successful in promoting community-based responses to stigma. Their influence can be extended to other issues as well. Survivors are just as comfortable reaching out to local leaders to confront stigma as they are seeking assistance to address problems in their families, jobs, and other aspects of their community. As brokers of change, community leaders can also be used to advance the welfare of the socially marginalized and complement the work of humanitarian organizations with similar objectives.

Societies, Inequality, and the Future of Epidemics

Barring dramatic improvements in living standards in developing countries, their weak health systems and underdeveloped systems of social support will continue to increase their exposure to future epidemics. African countries are particularly vulnerable to these events, not just because they host the majority of the world's poorest nations. Also relevant is the fact that most of them are in the early stages of the epidemiological transition. Scholars studying these transitions indicate that the major causes of death observed within countries change as they go through the process of economic development.[16] Accordingly, while non-infectious diseases such as cancers, cardiovascular disease, and respiratory diseases are among the major causes of death in the developed world, the major causes of death in poor African countries are infectious diseases such as cholera, measles, and pertussis.

By virtue of their fragile economic systems and current epidemiological profiles, African countries are among the most likely places where the social consequences of future epidemics will be observed. Widespread poverty in rural Africa and the ensuing increases in human contact with animals could lead to the spread of more zoonotic diseases that cause epidemics, just as seen at the start of the 2014 Ebola crisis. Some of these countries have already experienced outbreaks of disease, such as Crimean-Congo hemorrhagic fever and the Marburg virus, which have no known cures. Large outbreaks of such diseases could have similar long-term consequences for populations to those associated with Ebola. With recent improvements in global travel, the risks associated with the effects of these outbreaks will be felt beyond the borders of the countries where they started.

Social inequalities within countries will continue to shape the landscape around which these problems will occur. Unless attention is given to improving the welfare of people on the margins of society, they will continue to experience the brunt of these problems. Failing to improve their health systems will make it difficult to mount effective medical responses to the spread of diseases. Without the investments needed to improve the fragile social infrastructure of these countries, they will continue to carry the disproportionate burdens of tragedies such as family fragmentation and the loss of livelihoods. Many Ebola survivors still continue to live with the challenges created by these medical and social consequences, and it remains unclear what their recovery would eventually look like. One hopes it will involve an increase in their ability to return to the lives they had before the epidemic, although, at this point, many of them have fallen short of reaching this ideal. Nevertheless, there are reasons to remain hopeful.

Ebola survivors continue to take small steps to adapt to their current socioeconomic circumstances and make the best of what they have. Progress toward the goal of full recovery after epidemics should remain a priority for policymakers and NGOs. Complete recovery will be achieved only by making the investments needed to improve lives after epidemics.

Acknowledgments

I thank God for all the things that had to come together for me to successfully complete this project. I started planning to study the experiences of Ebola survivors in West Africa almost immediately after completing my book on the 2014 Ebola outbreak in Dallas, Texas. However, it took two attempts for these plans to be translated into reality. The first occurred in early 2020, after I received a small grant from the Center for Global Studies at Pennsylvania State University to study the lives of Ebola survivors. However, my plan to travel to West Africa to begin the project was subsequently derailed by the start of the COVID-19 pandemic. Later that year, I moved to the University of Texas at Austin, where I made a second attempt to kickstart the project. Based on another proposal I developed for studying the lives of Ebola survivors, the university nominated me for the Carnegie Fellowship, which I subsequently received. This fellowship provided generous funds that supported my fieldwork in Liberia and Sierra Leone.

While in these countries, I met with several individuals who were instrumental to the success of this project. The most important were the many Ebola survivors who agreed to be interviewed, voluntarily shared their experiences with the disease, and discussed how they have fared since the end of the 2014 epidemic. A few of them were initially reluctant to participate in the process because they had been interviewed so many times in the past by others interested in the epidemic. Other survivors simply wanted someone to talk to. They wanted to have their voices heard and let others know how they had overcome their tragic experiences. After participating in the interviews, many survivors helped to spread the word about the project, which provided opportunities for conducting more interviews.

Critical to the success of the project was the work of two small research teams I recruited to help conduct fieldwork in Liberia and Sierra Leone. The team in Liberia included Reginald Gbedee and Richlue Morris, while that in Sierra Leone included Bisolu Betts and Titus Alpha. After being informed about the goals of the project and receiving training to conduct the interviews, they helped to identify potential respondents, arrange appointments, and conduct interviews with Ebola survivors. I trusted them as we walked through crowded neighborhoods to interview respondents, shared rides on *kehkehs*, and as they used their social networks and experiences to advance the goals of the project. For example, Titus Alpha used his experience with a nongovernmental organization (NGO) working with Ebola survivors in rural areas to conduct interviews with survivors in villages in Sierra Leone's Moyamba district. Richlue Morris used his prior experience as a volunteer at an Ebola Treatment Unit in Liberia during the epidemic to provide additional perspective on how Ebola patients were cared for during this period. Additionally, Bisolu Betts in Sierra Leone used his many contacts in Freetown to track down survivors in some of the most marginalized communities.

The project also benefited from the assistance of several government officials and leaders of Ebola survivor organizations in Liberia and Sierra Leone. Gloria Mason and staff of the National Research Ethics Board, based at the John F. Kennedy hospital in Monrovia, Liberia, provided vital assistance needed for securing ethics approval for the project in Liberia. Edward Foday and his team at the Sierra Leone Ethics and Scientific Review Committee provided similar assistance for doing fieldwork in Sierra Leone. I am also grateful for assistance received from Anthony Naileh and members of the executive committee of the National Ebola Survivors Network of Liberia, who shared their perspectives with me and provided access to an extended network of Ebola survivors in the country. The national leader of Sierra Leone's Ebola Survivors Association, Yusuf Kabba, and other local leaders of the association were equally helpful. In fact, some of them even allowed us to use space in the association's premises to conduct interviews with some Ebola survivors.

Some of the work presented in this book was inspired by conversations I had with scholars and students around my general interest in the Ebola epidemic. These include my former colleagues at Pennsylvania State University and my former colleagues at the University of Texas at Austin. I was fortunate to receive feedback on various aspects of the project from students and scholars during two presentations I gave on selected issues in the study. The first was a presentation entitled "The 2014 Ebola Epidemic and Its Consequences in the United States and West Africa" that was part of the speaker series on Humanities, Health, and Medicine, at the University of Texas at Austin. The second was a presentation entitled "The Social Consequences of Surviving Epidemics: Ebola Survivors and Their Return to Community Life in Liberia and Sierra Leone" given at the International Conference on Medical Humanities at Birkbeck College, University of London.

I also want to acknowledge the efforts of Robin Coleman and the staff of Johns Hopkins University Press for working with me through every stage of the publication of this book. They were diligent in getting the manuscript through the review process and were responsive to my questions and concerns. Overall, the assistance I received from them was nothing but remarkable.

My wife, Tina, and daughters, Abigail and Lydia, were particularly charitable with their kindness and understanding as I worked on the project. Doing fieldwork in Liberia and Sierra Leone required frequent travel. In many cases, I did this without them. In my absence, Tina did double duty to take care of the family. However, it was always good to return home to Texas and share my experiences with them. Apart from this, being home allowed me to resume doing the things I needed to do as a husband and dad to keep myself grounded.

While working in Sierra Leone, where I was born, I was privileged to be around my parents, Jeremiah and Floretta Thomas, who are among my biggest cheerleaders and major sources of inspiration. They always wanted to know what they could do to help make the project successful and took their offers seriously. At almost 80 years of age, my dad, who had read my previous books, was particularly invested in seeing this one completed. In fact, before I started fieldwork, he regularly went to the archives of Sierra Leone's Independent Media Commission to find old newspaper articles about the Ebola epidemic that he thought I could use for the project. Toward the end of my fieldwork his health dramatically declined. However, this did not dissuade him from trying to be involved. Indeed, while he was on an oxygen machine, he volunteered to transcribe some of the interviews and translate them into English. Unfortunately, he took his final breath before the project was concluded. This book is dedicated to his memory. There are no words to express the value of the investments my dad made in me.

Chapter 1. Beginning Life at the End of Epidemics

1. Like all other Ebola survivors interviewed for the study, this individual is identified using a pseudonym to protect his identity.

2. These numbers are taken from estimates provided by the Centers for Disease Control and Prevention, "2014–2016 Ebola Outbreak in West Africa," March 8, 2019, https://www.cdc.gov/vhf/ebola/history/2014-2016-outbreak /index.html. The number of survivors is estimated as the number of reported cases minus the number of reported deaths in each country.

3. Barr and Podolsky, "National Medical Response to Crisis."

4. Green, "West African Countries Focus."

5. The new vaccines that have been approved are the rVSV-ZEBOV, Zabdeno/ Mvabea, and Ad5-EBOV vaccines.

6. Ideally, a thorough analysis of the lives of Ebola survivors would require the use of extensive demographic data collected in a census of all survivors. Unfortunately, such data are not available; but even if they were, they would be limited in their ability to provide the kind of in-depth analysis that could be done with information collected from the type of qualitative data this study collected from Ebola survivors.

7. This sample was added after my serendipitous meeting with someone who previously worked with survivors in that area and was fluent in the language spoken in that region. This person worked as a research assistant for the project and was instrumental in collecting the narratives from interviews conducted in this region.

8. Index Mundi, "Liberia vs. Sierra Leone."

9. For more extensive discussion, see Hays, *Epidemics and Pandemics*, 1–8.

10. Frankel, "Imagine a Disease Wiping Out."

11. Centers for Disease Control and Prevention, "2014–2016 Ebola Outbreak."

12. World Bank, "Physicians (per 1,000 People)."

13. Mullan, "The Cost of Ebola," e423.

14. Takahashi et al., "Reduced Vaccination."

15. Ribacke et al., "The Impact of the West Africa Ebola Outbreak."

16. Leuenberger et al., "Impact of the Ebola Epidemic on General and HIV Care."

17. Leach, "The Ebola Crisis and Post-2015 Development," 818.

18. This percentage is derived from the estimated number of infections and total deaths for Guinea, Liberia, and Sierra Leone provided by the CDC.

19. See, for example, the description of how trauma lived on in the memories of survivors of the 1918 flu pandemic in Davis, "The Forgotten Apocalypse."

20. Bristow, "'It's as Bad as Anything Can Be,'" 137.

21. Porter, "The Patient's View," 174.

22. Snyder et al., "Ebola in Urban Slums."

23. For more information, see Dols, *The Black Death in the Middle East.*"

24. Peters, *Smallpox in the New World*, 12.

25. Riedel, "Edward Jenner and the History," 21.

26. This perspective is presented and challenged by Tierney and Oliver-Smith, who acknowledge the prior tendency to define recovery as a return to the *status quo ante* but argue that the process is now used to refer to a movement toward the new normal. More discussion is found in Tierney and Oliver-Smith, "Social Dimensions of Disaster Recovery."

27. Government of Sierra Leone, *National Ebola Recovery Strategy.*

28. Fofana and Bavier, "Ebola Victims Sue Sierra Leone."

29. Zapotoczny, "The Political and Social Consequences."

30. Herring, "'There Were Young People,'" 87.

31. For more discussion, see Dobyns, *Their Number Become Thinned.*

32. Gamsa, "The Epidemic of Pneumonic Plague," 163.

33. For more information, see Dols, *The Black Death in the Middle East.*

34. Zapotoczny, "The Political and Social Consequences."

35. Zapotoczny, "The Political and Social Consequences."

36. Garret, "We Did It."

37. Reuters Staff, "DRC: Last Ebola Patient."

38. Ryan and Walsh, "Consequences of Non-Intervention."

39. Genton et al., "Recovery Potential of a Western Lowland Gorilla Population."

40. Genton et al., "Recovery Potential of a Western Lowland Gorilla Population."

41. Matua and Locsin, "Conquering Death from Ebola."

42. Matua and Locsin, "Conquering Death from Ebola."

43. Matua and Locsin, "Conquering Death from Ebola."

44. Delamou et al., "Profile and Reintegration Experience of Ebola Survivors," 254.

45. James et al., "Post-Ebola Psychosocial Experiences," 685.

46. Matua and Locsin, "Conquering Death from Ebola."

47. Matua and Locsin, "Conquering Death from Ebola."

48. Van Griensven et al., "Evaluation of Convalescent Plasma."

49. Epstein et al., "Infectious Disease: Mobilizing Ebola Survivors."

50. Stein et al., "To Hasten Ebola Containment, Mobilize Survivors," 1679.

51. Farbu et al., "Polio Survivors," 500.

Chapter 2. Social Determinants of Recovery

1. These announcements belied the fact that the end of the Ebola epidemic was a gradual process. In Liberia, the virus re-emerged at least three times after the first announcement of the end of the epidemic. Similarly, there were multiple announcements of the end of the epidemics in Guinea and Sierra Leone. However, the outbreaks in these countries officially ended before those in Liberia.

2. World Health Organization, "End of the Most Recent Ebola Virus."

3. Richards, *Ebola. How a People's Science.*

4. For example, during the HIV/AIDS epidemic, the most affected groups in many countries were sex workers, men having sex with men (MSM), and people experiencing poverty.

5. Snyder et al, "Ebola in Urban Slums."

6. Cacioppo, "Build Your Social Resilience."

7. Masten and Obradovic, "Disaster Preparation and Recovery," 8.

8. Masten and Obradovic, "Disaster Preparation and Recovery," 9.

9. Rabelo et al., "Psychological Distress among Ebola Survivors."

10. Schwerdtle et al., "Experiences of Ebola Survivors."

11. Bonanno et al., "Psychological Resilience and Dysfunction."

12. Farber et al., "Resilience Factors Associated with Adaptation."

13. Maddi, "Personal Hardiness as the Basis for Resilience."

14. Keating and Hanger-Kopp, "Practitioner Perspectives of Disaster."

15. Keating and Hanger-Koop, "Practitioner Perspectives of Disaster," 3.

16. Nigg, *Disaster Recovery as a Social Process.*

17. Onyango et al., "Gender-Based Violence."

18. Greenlees et al., "From the Great Plague to the 1918 Flu."

19. Greenlees et al., "From the Great Plague to the 1918 Flu."

20. Kumar et al., "Corona Pandemic and Disruption in Social Structure."

21. Richards et al., "Social Pathways for Ebola Virus."

22. James et al., "An Assessment of Ebola-Related Stigma."

23. Kumar et al., "Corona Pandemic and Disruption in Social Structure," 3.

24. Virk, "Victim or Advocate?"

25. Collins, "The Political Ecology of Hazard Vulnerability."

26. Reid, "Disasters and Social Inequalities," 984.

27. Barde, "Plague in San Francisco."

28. Markel, "Knocking Out Cholera."

29. See, for example, Gage et al., "Defining Learning Loss."

30. Kapiriri and Ross, "The Politics of Disease Epidemics."

31. There is some overlap between the place of residence and social class, given that, on average rural residents are more likely to be considered members of the lower class, while urban areas are where most members of the upper class reside.

32. Stock, *Africa South of the Sahara*, 241.

33. Farmer, *Fevers, Feuds, and Diamonds.*

34. Fabricant et al., "Why the Poor Pay More," 184.

35. Macrotrends, "Monrovia, Liberia Metro Area Population."

36. Macrotrends, "Freetown, Sierra Leone Metro Area Population."

37. Abdullah, "Bush Path to Destruction."

38. MacDougall, "Fearing the Tide in West Point."

39. Summers et al., "Challenges in Responding to the Ebola Epidemic."

40. Summers et al., "Challenges in Responding to the Ebola Epidemic."

41. Richards et al., "Social Pathways for Ebola Virus."

42. Frankfurter, "Discerning Epidemic Preparedness in Sierra Leone."

43. Reid, "Disasters and Social Inequalities."

44. Benton and Dionne, "International Political Economy."

45. Boseley, "Experts Criticize WHO Delay."

46. More discussion on this is found in Hall and Michele Lamont, "Why Social Relations Matter."

47. Obeng-Odoom and Bockarie, "The Political Economy of the Ebola Virus."

48. Missoni, "The Political Economy of Epidemics."

49. In rare cases these resources can be marshaled in the absence of these traditions, as was observed during the mobilization efforts of Uganda's government to tackle the devastating effects of the HIV/AIDS epidemic in the 1990s.

50. Government of Sierra Leone, "National Ebola Recovery Strategy."

51. Cohen and Werker, "The Political Economy of 'Natural' Disasters," 795–96.

52. Cohen and Werker, "The Political Economy of 'Natural' Disasters," 796.

53. Obeng-Odoom and Bockarie, "The Political Economy of the Ebola Virus."

54. Onwujekwe et al., "Corruption in Anglophone West Africa Health Systems," 531–32.

55. Lee-Jones et al., "Liberia: Overview of Corruption and Anti-Corruption," 5.

56. Root, "After Ebola Funds Fiasco."

Chapter 3. Family Life in the Aftermath of Ebola

1. Shehu, "Social Police Regarding the Transformation of Family."

2. Farmer, *Fevers, Feuds, and Diamonds*, 101.

3. Jensen et al., *Perpetrators and Protectors.*"

4. McFerson, "Women and Post-Conflict Society in Sierra Leone."

5. Horn et al., "'I Don't Need an Eye for an Eye.'"

6. Godwin, "Understanding the Reproductive Health."

7. Richardson et al., "The Ebola Suspect's Dilemma."

8. Richards, *Ebola*.

9. See, for example, Matua and Van der Wal, "Living Under the Constant Threat of Ebola," and Arwady et al., "Reintegration of Ebola Survivors," 1207.

10. Taylor et al., "Fictive Kin Networks."

11. Peterman, "Widowhood and Asset Inheritance."

12. United Nations News Center, "West African Communities Receiving Ebola's Orphans."

13. Inhofe, "A Call to Support Those Orphaned."

14. Evans and Popova, "Orphans and Ebola."

15. Martin, *Mapping of Residential Care Institutions*.

16. S.O.S. Children's Villages, "General Information on Sierra Leone."

17. "Liberian Orphanages."

18. One US dollar was equal to about 10,000 leones at the time of the study.

19. Case et al., "Orphans in Africa."

20. "Sierra Leone: Grant-in-Aid Award."

Chapter 4. The Health Consequences of Prior Ebola Infection

1. Gulland, "Thousands of Ebola Survivors."

2. Cunha, "The Cause of the Plague of Athens."

3. Battles and Gilmour, "Beyond Mortality: Survivors of Epidemic Infections."

4. Efstathiou et al., "Suicidality and COVID-19."

5. Inciardi and Chandra, "Long COVID-19," 18.

6. Mehtar et al., "Deliberate Exposure of Humans to Chlorine."

7. Secor et al., "Mental Health Among Ebola Survivors."

8. Yadav and Rawal, "The Current Mental Health Status," LA01.

9. Billioux et al., "Neurological Complications of Ebola."

10. Billioux et al., "Neurological Complications of Ebola."

11. The relationship between persistent dizziness, which is a mental health concern, and neurological problems is now well recognized in the literature. However, dizziness is also a symptom of other health conditions, such as infection or poor circulation.

12. Shantha et al., "An Update on Ocular Complications."

13. Shantha et al., "An Update on Ocular Complications."

14. National Institutes of Health, "Study Finds Ebola Survivors."

15. Partners in Health, "Blindness."

16. Partners in Health, "Blindness."

17. Grady, "Ebola's Legacy: Children with Cataracts."

18. Grady, "Ebola's Legacy: Children with Cataracts."

19. Kelland, "Thousands of Ebola Survivors Face Severe Pain."

20. Wilson et al., "Post-Ebola Syndrome."

21. Scott et al., "Post-Ebola Syndrome, Sierra Leone."

22. Wilson et al., "Post-Ebola Syndrome."

23. Wilson et al., "Post-Ebola Syndrome."

24. Godwin et al., "Reproductive Health Sequelae Among Women."

25. Godwin et al., "Reproductive Health Sequelae Among Women."

26. Farmer, *Fevers, Feuds, and Diamonds.*

27. Farmer, *Fevers, Feuds, and Diamonds.*

28. Among the concerns expressed by Liberian survivors was the fear that they were being used as guinea pigs for medical studies. There were also minor concerns about the effectiveness of the treatment that were receiving. Some survivors, for example, wanted to receive something other than basic painkillers for their chronic pains.

29. In general, some of the limitations are discussed in Omonzejele, "Current Ethical and Other Problems."

30. Steptoe et al., "Visual Disability in Ebola Survivors."

31. World Health Organization, "Improving Access to Mental Health Services."

32. Doctors Without Borders, "Liberia: Providing Psychiatric Care."

Chapter 5. The Stickiness of Stigma

1. Kelly et al., "Ebola Virus Disease-Related Stigma."

2. Secor et al., "Mental Health Among Ebola Survivors."

3. Choi, " 'People Look at Me Like I AM the Virus.' "

4. Very few systematic studies exist on the stigma of COVID-19 among patients in the United States. However, the overall prevalence of COVID-19 stigma was very low at the height of the pandemic, estimated to have been experienced by only 3% of the U.S. population. More information can be found in Gutierrez et al., "Experiences of Stigma in the United States."

5. Overholt et al., "Stigma and Ebola Survivorship in Liberia."

6. A great synopsis of these programs can be found in Brown et al., "Interventions to Reduce HIV/AIDS Stigma."

7. Long, "Fighting Fear and Stigma."

8. Long, "Fighting Fear and Stigma."

9. See, for example, Denis-Ramirez et al., "In the Midst of a 'Perfect Storm.' "

10. Goffman, *Stigma*, 11.

11. A useful description of the relationship among stigma, labeling, and social class is found in Link and Phelan, "Conceptualizing Stigma."

12. Van Bortel et al., "Psychosocial Effects of an Ebola Outbreak."

13. Denis-Ramirez et al., "In the Midst of a 'Perfect Storm.' "

14. Long, "Fighting Fear and Stigma."

15. This was approximately $11 at that time.

16. Crea et al., "Social Distancing, Community Stigma, and Implications."

17. Crea et al., "Social Distancing, Community Stigma, and Implications."

18. The use of these narratives was widespread in both Liberia and Sierra Leone. See, for example, Mayrhuber et al., " 'We Are Survivors and Not a Virus.' "

19. Butler-Warke, "There's a Time and a Place."

20. Alenichev, " 'We Will Soon Be Dead.' "

21. Alenichev, " 'We Will Soon Be Dead.' "

Chapter 6. Livelihood Strategies and the Economic Consequences of the Epidemic

1. Connolly, *Communicable Disease Control in Emergencies.*

2. Ojha, "Is Pandemic a Class-Ridden?"

3. Keogh-Brown, "Macroeconomic Effect of Infectious Disease."

4. Lewis, "The Economics of Epidemics."

5. Government of Sierra Leone, "National Ebola Recovery Strategy."

6. White et al., *African Poverty at the Millennium.*

7. Bausch and Schwarz, "Outbreak of Ebola Virus Disease in Guinea."

8. Neufeld, "Hygiene Conditions in Ancient Israel."

9. Echenberg, "Pestis Redux."

10. Sutmoller et al., "Control and Eradication of Foot-and-Mouth."

11. Echenberg, "Pestis Redux."

12. Connolly, "Communicable Disease Control in Emergencies."

13. Kinsman, "A Time of Fear."

14. Rabelo et al., "Psychological Distress Among Ebola Survivors."

15. Sindzingre, "Theoretical Criticisms and Policy Optimism."

16. Audet, "From Disaster Relief to Development Assistance."

17. Momoh was referred to the fieldwork team by locals who identified him as the person one needed to contact for help recruiting Ebola survivors for the interviews. He helped us gain access to his community and identify other potential interview subjects, who were screened to determine whether they met the eligibility requirements for the interview.

18. National Public Radio, "The Ebola Survivors Who Can't Go Home."

19. The specific amounts stated by survivors varied, but most reported cash payments of 500,000 to 750,000 Leones, which was between $50 and $75 at the time they received these payments.

20. Other names for the same practice include *esusu* (Nigeria), *tontines* (Senegal), and *janji* (Cameroon). See Center for Development and Security Excellence, "Potential Risk in Informal Banking and Finance Job Aid."

21. This frustration was also expressed by those who were skeptical of participating in this study. The response they received involved first acknowl-

edging their frustrations. Thereafter, they were told that the primary purpose of the study is to advance research, which could provide a basis for developing interventions to address these issues.

22. Root, "After Ebola Funds Fiasco."

Chapter 7. Beyond Medical Responses

1. Banauch et al., "Pulmonary Disease in Rescue Workers."
2. Bergen, "September 11 Attacks: United States."
3. Neria et al., "Mental and Physical Health Consequences."
4. Moncivais, "911 Victims Compensation."
5. Moncivais, "911 Victims Compensation."
6. Keith, "Final Coverage Provisions."
7. Congress.gov, "H.R.98 - COVID-19 Victims Compensation Fund Act."
8. See, for example, Feinberg, "The September 11th Victim Compensation Fund." The $7 billion estimate excludes the cost of subsequent expansions to compensate other victims of the September 11 attacks.
9. Chang et al., "Phase- and Epidemic Region-Adjusted Estimation."
10. NBC News, "Why Has Nurse Amber Vinson Recovered?"
11. African Development Bank Group, "Sierra Leone: $13.5 Million Project."
12. Social Security Administration, "Liberia."
13. International Labor Organization, "Sierra Leone."
14. Han and Curtis, "Social Responses to Epidemics."
15. KFF, "The U.S. President's Emergency Plan."
16. Santosa et al., "The Development and Experience."

Works Cited

Abdullah, Ibrahim. "Bush Path to Destruction: The Origin and Character of the Revolutionary United Front/Sierra Leone." *Journal of Modern African Studies* 36, no. 2 (June 1998): 203–35. https://doi.org/10.1017/S0022278X98002766.

African Development Bank Group. "Sierra Leone: $13.5 Million Project to Assist Ebola-Hit Communities Kicks Off." 2020. https://www.afdb.org/en/news-and -events/press-releases/sierra-leone-135-million-project-assist-ebola-hit -communities-kicks-37302.

Alenichev, Arsenii. "'We Will Soon Be Dead': Stigma and Cascades of Looping Effects in a Collaborative Ebola Vaccine Trial." *Critical Public Health* 31, no. 1 (2021): 55–65. https://doi.org/10.1080/09581596.2019.1682124.

Arwady, M. Allison, Edmundo L. Garcia, Benedict Wollor, Lyndon G. Mabande, Erik J. Reaves, and Joel M. Montgomery. "Reintegration of Ebola survivors into Their Communities—Firestone District, Liberia, 2014." *Morbidity and Mortality Weekly Report* 63, no. 50 (2014): 1207–9. https://www.cdc.gov/mmwr /preview/mmwrhtml/mm6350a7.htm?s_cid=mm6350a7_w.

Audet, François. "From Disaster Relief to Development Assistance: Why Simple Solutions Don't Work." *International Journal* 70, no. 1 (2015): 110–18. https:// doi.org/10.1177/0020702014562595.

Banauch, Gisela I., Atiya Dhala, and David J. Prezant. "Pulmonary Disease in Rescue Workers at the World Trade Center Site." *Current Opinion in Pulmonary Medicine* 11, no. 2 (2005): 160–68. https://doi.org/10.1097/01.mcp .0000151716.96241.0a.

Barde, Robert. "Plague in San Francisco: An Essay Review." *Journal of the History of Medicine and Allied Sciences* 59, no. 3 (2004): 463–70. https://doi.org/10 .1093/jhmas/jrh104.

Barr, Justin, and Scott H. Podolsky. "A National Medical Response to Crisis— The Legacy of World War II." *New England Journal of Medicine* 383, no. 7 (2020): 613–15. https://doi.org/10.1056/NEJMp2008512.

Battles, Heather, and Rebecca Gilmour. "Beyond Mortality: Survivors of Epidemic Infections and the Bioarchaeology of Impairment and Disability."

Bioarchaeology International 6, no. 1–2 (2022): 23–40. https://doi.org/10.5744 /bi.2021.0003.

Bausch, Daniel G., and Lara Schwarz. "Outbreak of Ebola Virus Disease in Guinea: Where Ecology Meets Economy." *PLoS Neglected Tropical Diseases* 8, no. 7 (2014): e3056. https://doi.org/10.1371/journal.pntd.0003056.

Benton, Adia, and Kim Yi Dionne. "International Political Economy and the 2014 West African Ebola Outbreak." *African Studies Review* 58, no. 1 (March 2015): 223–36. https://doi.org/10.1017/asr.2015.11.

Bergen, Peter. "September 11 Attacks: United States." Britannica.com. 2023. https://www.britannica.com/event/September-11-attacks.

Billioux, Bridgette Jeanne, Bryan Smith, and Avindra Nath, "Neurological Complications of Ebola Virus Infection." *Neurotherapeutics* 13, no. 3 (July 2016): 461–70. https://doi.org/10.1007/s13311–016–0457–z.

Bonanno, George A., Samuel M. Y. Ho, Jane C. K. Chan, et al. "Psychological Resilience and Dysfunction Among Hospitalized Survivors of the SARS Epidemic in Hong Kong: A Latent Class Approach." *Health Psychology* 27, no. 5 (2008). https://doi.org/10.1037/0278–6133.27.5.659.

Boseley, Sarah. "Experts Criticise WHO Delay in Sounding Alarm over Ebola Outbreak." *Guardian*, November 22, 2015. https://www.theguardian.com /world/2015/nov/22/experts-criticise-world-health-organisation-who-delay -ebola-outbreak.

Bristow, Nancy K. "'It's as Bad as Anything Can Be': Patients, Identity, and the Influenza Pandemic." Supplement, *Public Health Reports* 125, no. 3 (2010): 134–44. https://doi.org/10.1177/00333549101250S316.

Brown, Lisanne, Kate Macintyre, and Lea Trujillo. "Interventions to Reduce HIV/AIDS Stigma: What Have We Learned?" *AIDS Education and Prevention* 15, no. 1 (2003): 49–69. https://doi.org/10.1521/aeap.15.1.49.23844.

Butler-Warke, Alice. "There's a Time and a Place: Temporal Aspects of Place-Based Stigma." *Community Development Journal* 56, no. 2 (2021): 203–19. https://doi.org/10.1093/cdj/bsaa040.

Cacioppo, John. "Build Your Social Resilience: Would You Like to Build Your Social Resilience? *Psychology Today Blog*, March 6, 2020. https://www .psychologytoday.com/us/blog/connections/201003/build-your-social -resilience.

Case, Anne, Christina Paxson, and Joseph Ableidinger. "Orphans in Africa: Parental Death, Poverty, and School Enrollment." *Demography* 41, no. 3 (2004): 483–508. https://doi.org/10.1353/dem.2004.0019.

Center for Development and Security Excellence. "Potential Risk in Informal Banking and Finance Job Aid." Accessed June 2023. https://www.cdse.edu /Portals/124/Documents/jobaids/insider/Potential-Risk-in-Informal-Banking .pdf.

Centers for Disease Control and Prevention. "2014–2016 Ebola Outbreak in West Africa." Accessed July 1, 2023. https://www.cdc.gov/vhf/ebola/history/2014 -2016-outbreak/index.html.

Chang, Ruijie, Huwen Wang, Shuxian Zhang, et al. "Phase- and Epidemic Region-Adjusted Estimation of the Number of Coronavirus Disease 2019 Cases in China." *Frontiers of Medicine* 14, no. 2 (March 2020): 199–209. https://doi .org/10.1007/s11684-020-0768-7.

Choi, Shinwoo. " 'People Look at Me Like I AM the Virus': Fear, Stigma, and Discrimination During the COVID-19 Pandemic." *Qualitative Social Work* 20, no. 1–2 (2021): 233–39. https://doi.org/10.1177/1473325020973333.

Cohen, Charles, and Eric D. Werker. "The Political Economy of Natural Disasters." *Journal of Conflict Resolution* 52, no. 6 (2008): 795–819. https://doi.org /10.1177/0022002708322157.

Collins, Timothy W. "The Political Ecology of Hazard Vulnerability: Marginalization, Facilitation and the Production of Differential Risk to Urban Wildfires in Arizona's White Mountains." *Journal of Political Ecology* 15, no. 1 (2008): 21–43. https://doi.org/10.2458/v15i1.21686.

Congress.gov. "H.R.98 - COVID-19 Victims Compensation Fund Act." 2021. https://www.congress.gov/bill/117th-congress/house-bill/98/text.

Connolly, Máire A. *Communicable Disease Control in Emergencies: A Field Manual.* World Health Organization, 2005. https://www.who.int/publi cations/i/item/communicable-disease-control-in-emergencies-a-field -manual.

Crea, Thomas M., K. Megan Collier, Elizabeth K. Klein, et al. "Social Distancing, Community Stigma, and Implications for Psychological Distress in the Aftermath of Ebola Virus Disease." *PLoS ONE* 17, no. 11 (2022): e0276790. https://doi.org/10.1371/journal.pone.0276790.

Cunha, Burke. "The Cause of the Plague of Athens: Plague, Typhoid, Typhus, Smallpox, or Measles?" *Infectious Disease Clinics* 18, no. 1 (March 2004): 29–43. https://doi.org/10.1016/S0891-5520(03)00100-4.

Davis, David. "The Forgotten Apocalypse: Katherine Anne Porter's 'Pale Horse, Pale Rider,' Traumatic Memory, and the Influenza Pandemic of 1918." *Southern Literary Journal* 43, no. 2 (2011): 55–74. https://dx.doi.org/10.1353/slj .2011.0007

Delamou, Alexandre, Bienvenu Salim Camara, Jean Pe Kolie, et al. "Profile and Reintegration Experience of Ebola Survivors in Guinea: A Cross-Sectional Study." *Tropical Medicine & International Health* 22, no. 3 (2017): 254–60. https://doi.org/10.1111/tmi.12825

Denis-Ramirez, Elise, Katrine Holmegaard Sørensen, and Morten Skovdal. "In the Midst of a 'Perfect Storm': Unpacking the Causes and Consequences of Ebola-Related Stigma for Children Orphaned by Ebola in Sierra Leone."

Children and Youth Services Review 73 (2017): 445–53. https://doi.org/10.1016
/j.childyouth.2016.11.025.

Dobyns, Henry. *Their Number Become Thinned: Native American Population
Dynamics in Eastern North America.* University of Tennessee Press, 1983.

Doctors Without Borders. "Liberia: Providing Psychiatric Care Close to Home."
July 2019. https://www.doctorswithoutborders.org/latest/liberia-providing
-psychiatric-care-close-home.

Dols, Michael Walters. *The Black Death in the Middle East.* Princeton University
Press, 2019.

Echenberg, Myron. "Pestis Redux: The Initial Years of the Third Bubonic Plague
Pandemic, 1894–1901." *Journal of World History* 13, no. 2 (2002): 429–49.
https://www.jstor.org/stable/20078978.

Efstathiou, Vasiliki, Maria-Ioanna Stefanou, Nikolaos Siafakas, et al. "Suicidality
and COVID19: Suicidal Ideation, Suicidal Behaviors and Completed Suicides
Amidst the COVID19 Pandemic." *Experimental and Therapeutic Medicine* 23,
no. 1 (2022): 1–8. https://doi.org/10.3892/etm.2021.11030.

Epstein, Joshua M., Lauren M. Sauer, Julia Chelen, et al. "Infectious Disease:
Mobilizing Ebola Survivors to Curb the Epidemic." *Nature News* 516, no. 7531
(2014): 323. https://doi.org/10.1038/516323a y.

Evans, David and Anna Popova. "Orphans and Ebola: Estimating the Secondary
Impact of a Public Health Crisis." *World Bank Policy Research Working Paper*
7196 (2015). https://papers.ssrn.com/sol3/papers.cfm?abstract_id=2579891#.

Fabricant, Stephen J., Clifford W. Kamara, and Anne Mills. "Why the Poor Pay
More: Household Curative Expenditures in Rural Sierra Leone." *International
Journal of Health Planning and Management* 14, no. 3 (1999): 179–99. https://
doi.org/10.1002/(SICI)1099–1751(199907/09)14:3%3C179::AID-HPM548
%3E3.0.CO;2-N.

Farber, Eugene W., Jennifer A. J. Schwartz, Paul E. Schaper, DeElla J. Moonen,
and J. Stephen McDaniel. "Resilience Factors Associated with Adaptation to
HIV Disease." *Psychosomatics* 41, no. 2 (2000): 140–46. https://doi.org/10.1176
/appi.psy.41.2.140.

Farbu, Elisabeth, Tiina Rekand, Johan A. Aarli, and Nils Erik Gilhus. "Polio
Survivors—Well Educated and Hard Working." *Journal of Neurology* 248,
no. 6 (2001): 500–505. https://doi.org/10.1007/s004150170160.

Farmer, Paul. *Fevers, Feuds, and Diamonds: Ebola and the Ravages of History.*
Farrar, Straus and Giroux, 2020.

Feinberg, Kenneth R. "The September 11th Victim Compensation Fund of 2001:
Policy and Precedent." *New York Law School Law Review* 56, no. 3 (January
2012): 1115–18. https://heinonline.org/HOL/LandingPage?handle=hein
.journals/nyls56&div=45&id=&page=.

Fofana, Umaru, and Joe Bavier. "Ebola Victims Sue Sierra Leone Government

Over Mismanaged Funds." Reuters. December 15, 2017. https://www.reuters
.com/article/us-health-ebola-leone/ebola-victims-sue-sierra-leone-govern
ment-over-mismanaged-funds-idUSKBN1E92NE.

Frankel, Todd. "Imagine a Disease Wiping Out 64,000 U.S. Doctors. Now, You
Understand Ebola in Sierra Leone." *Washington Post*, December 22, 2014.
https://www.washingtonpost.com/news/storyline/wp/2014/12/22/imagine
-a-disease-wiping-out-63000-u-s-doctors-now-you-understand-ebola-in
-sierra-leone/.

Frankfurter, Raphael. "Discerning Epidemic Preparedness in Sierra Leone."
Medical Anthropology 40, no.8 (2021): 699–702. https://doi.org/10.1080
/01459740.2021.1961250.

Gage, Nicholas, Ashley MacSuga-Gage, William Crawley, and Timothy E. Morse.
"Defining Learning Loss in Relation to the COVID-19 Pandemic." *Preventing
School Failure: Alternative Education for Children and Youth* 67, no. 3 (April
2023): 1–6. https://doi.org/10.1080/1045988X.2023.2204826.

Gamsa, Mark. "The Epidemic of Pneumonic Plague in Manchuria 1910–1911."
Past & Present 190, no. 1 (2006): 147–83. https://doi.org/10.1093/pastj/gtj001.

Garret, Laurie. "We Did It. We Beat the Virus." *Newsday*, May 31, 1995. https://
www.pulitzer.org/winners/laurie-garrett.

Genton, Celine, Romane Cristescu, Sylvain Gatti, et al. "Recovery Potential of
a Western Lowland Gorilla Population Following a Major Ebola Outbreak:
Results From a Ten-Year Study." *PLoS One* 7, no. 5 (2012): e37106. https://doi
.org/10.1371/journal.pone.0037106.

Godwin, Christine. "Understanding the Reproductive Health and Relationship
Changes of Women Who Survived Ebola in Liberia." PhD diss., University
of North Carolina at Chapel Hill, 2018. https://www.proquest.com/docview
/2060750887?fromopenview=true&pq-origsite=gscholar&sourcetype
=Dissertations%20&%20Theses.

Godwin, Christine L., David A. Wohl, William A. Fischer 2nd, et al. "Reproductive Health Sequelae Among Women Who Survived Ebola Virus Disease in
Liberia." *International Journal of Gynecology & Obstetrics* 146, no. 2 (2019):
212–17. https://doi.org/10.1002/ijgo.12858.

Goffman, Erving. *Stigma: Notes on the Management of Spoiled Identity.* Penguin
Books, 1963.

Government of Sierra Leone. "National Ebola Recovery Strategy for Sierra
Leone: 2015–2017." July 2015. https://ebolaresponse.un.org/sites/default/files
/sierra_leone_recovery_strategy_en.pdf.

Grady, Denise. "Ebola's Legacy: Children with Cataracts." *New York Times*,
November 19, 2017. https://www.nytimes.com/2017/10/19/health/ebola
-survivors-cataracts.html.

Green, Andrew. "West African Countries Focus on Post-Ebola Recovery Plans."

Lancet 388, no. 10059 (2016): 2463–65. https://doi.org/10.1016/S0140–6736 (16)32219-X.

Greenlees, Janet, Andrea Ford, and Sara Read. "From the Great Plague to the 1918 Flu, History Shows That Disease Outbreaks Make Inequality Worse." The Conversation. June 2021. https://theconversation.com/from-the-great -plague-to-the-1918-flu-history-shows-that-disease-outbreaks-make -inequality-worse-161945.

Gulland, Anne. "Thousands of Ebola Survivors Experience Serious Medical Complications." BMJ, 351 (2015): h4336. https://doi.org/10.1136/bmj.h4336.

Gutierrez, Amanda M., Sophie C. Schneider, Rubaiya Islam, et al. "Experiences of Stigma in the United States During the COVID-19 Pandemic." *Stigma and Health* (2022). https://doi.org/10.1037/sah0000354.

Hall, Peter, and Michele Lamont. "Why Social Relations Matter for Politics and Successful Societies." *Annual Review of Political Science* 16 (May 2013): 49–71. https://doi.org/10.1146/annurev-polisci-031710–101143.

Han, Qijun, and Daniel R. Curtis. "Social Responses to Epidemics Depicted by Cinema." *Emerging Infectious Diseases* 26, no. 2 (2020): 389–94. https://doi .org/10.3201/eid2602.181022.

Hays, Jo Nelson. *Epidemics and Pandemics: Their Impacts on Human History.* ABC-CLIO, 2005.

Herring, D. Ann. " 'There Were Young People and Old People and Babies Dying Every Week': The 1918–1919 Influenza Pandemic at Norway House." *Ethno- history* (1993): 73–105. https://doi.org/10.2307/3536979.

Horn, Rebecca, Eve S. Puffer, Elisabeth Roesch, and Heidi Lehmann. " 'I Don't Need an Eye for an Eye': Women's Responses to Intimate Partner Violence in Sierra Leone and Liberia." *Global Public Health* 11, no. 1–2 (2016): 108–21. https://doi.org/10.1080/17441692.2015.1032320.

Inciardi, Riccardo, and Alvin Chandra. "Long COVID-19: A Tangled Web of Lungs, Heart, Mind, and Gender." *Trends in Cardiovascular Medicine* 32, no. 1 (January 2022): 18–19. https://doi.org/10.1016/j.tcm.2021.10.004.

Index Mundi. "Liberia vs Sierra Leone." Accessed July 5, 2023. https://www .indexmundi.com/factbook/compare/liberia.sierra-leone.

Inhofe, Jim. "A Call to Support Those Orphaned by Ebola in West Africa." *Oklahoman*, May 2, 2015. https://www.oklahoman.com/story/opinion /columns/guest/2015/05/02/jim-inhofe-a-call-to-support-those-orphaned -by-ebola-in-west-africa/60749148007/.

International Labor Organization. "Sierra Leone." Accessed July 2023. https:// www.social-protection.org/gimi/ShowCountryProfile.action?iso=SL.

James, Peter Bai, Jonathan Wardle, Amie Steel, and Jon Adams. "An Assessment of Ebola-Related Stigma and Its Association with Informal Healthcare Utili- sation Among Ebola Survivors in Sierra Leone: A Cross-Sectional Study."

BMC Public Health 20, no. 1 (2020): 182. https://doi.org/10.1186/s12889
-020-8279-7.

James, Peter Bai, Jon Wardle, Amie Steel, and Jon Adams. "Post-Ebola Psychosocial Experiences and Coping Mechanisms Among Ebola Survivors: A
Systematic Review." *Tropical Medicine & International Health* 24, no. 6 (2019):
671–91. https://doi.org/10.1111/tmi.13226.

Jensen, Steffen Bo, Meghan Belcher, Juancho Reyes, Cartor Temba, Nohlanhla
Sibanda, and Dominique Dix Peek. *Perpetrators and Protectors: Centering
Family Relations in Addressing Violence in Poor Neighborhoods.* Dignity, the
Danish Institute against Torture, 2021.

Kapiriri, Lydia, and Alison Ross. "The Politics of Disease Epidemics: A Comparative Analysis of the SARS, Zika, and Ebola Outbreaks." *Global Social Welfare*
7, no. 1 (2020): 33–45. https://doi.org/10.1007/s40609-018-0123-y.

Keating, Adriana, and Susanne Hanger-Kopp. "Practitioner Perspectives of
Disaster Resilience in International Development." *International Journal of
Disaster Risk Reduction* 42 (2020): 101355. https://doi.org/10.1016/j.ijdrr.2019
.101355.

Keith, Katie. "Final Coverage Provisions in the American Rescue Plan and What
Comes Next." *Health Affairs Forefront,* 2021. https://www.healthaffairs.org
/content/forefront/final-coverage-provisions-american-rescue-plan-and
-comes-next.

Kelland, Kate. "Thousands of Ebola Survivors Face Severe Pain, Possible Blindness." Reuters. August 7, 2015. https://www.reuters.com/article/health-ebola
-survivors/thousands-of-ebola-survivors-face-severe-pain-possible-blindness
-idINKCN0QC1T720150807.

Kelly, J. Daniel, Sheri D. Weiser, Barthalomew Wilson, et al. "Ebola Virus
Disease-Related Stigma Among Survivors Declined in Liberia over an
18-Month, Post-Outbreak Period: An Observational Cohort Study." *PLoS
Neglected Tropical Diseases* 13, no. 2 (2019): e0007185. https://doi.org/10.1371
/journal.pntd.0007185.

Keogh-Brown, M. R. "Macroeconomic Effect of Infectious Disease Outbreaks."
Encyclopedia of Health Economics (2014): 177. https://doi.org/10.1016/B978
-0-12-375678-7.00608-8.

KFF. "The U.S. President's Emergency Plan for AIDS Relief (PEPFAR)." 2023.
https://www.kff.org/global-health-policy/fact-sheet/the-u-s-presidents
-emergency-plan-for-aids-relief-pepfar/.

Kinsman, John. "A Time of Fear": Local, National, and International Responses
to a Large Ebola Outbreak in Uganda." *Globalization and Health* 8 (2012):
1–12. https://doi.org/10.1186/1744-8603-8-15.

Kumar, Parveen, Kunzang Lamo, D. Namgyal, and Sonam Angchuck. "Corona
Pandemic and Disruption in Social Structure." *IOSR Journal of Humanities*

and Social Science 25, no. 6, Series 1 (June 2020): 23–25. https://doi.org/10
.9790/0837–2506012325.

Lamin, David F. M. "Mapping of Residential Care Institutions for Children in
Sierra Leone." UNICEF, 2008. https://bettercarenetwork.org/sites/default
/files/Mapping%20of%20Residential%20Care%20Institutions%20in%20
Sierra%20Leone.pdf.

Leach, Melissa. "The Ebola Crisis and Post-2015 Development." *Journal of
International Development* 27, no. 6 (2015): 816–34. https://doi.org/10.1002
/jid.3112.

Lee-Jones, Krista, R. M. B. Kukutschka, A. Miamen, and G. Nicaise. "Liberia:
Overview of Corruption and Anti-Corruption". *Transparency International*
(September 2019): 5. https://www.jstor.org/stable/pdf/resrep20503.pdf.

Leuenberger, David, Jean Hebelamou, Stefan Strahm, Nathalie De Rekeneire,
Eric Balestre, Gilles Wandeler, and François Dabis. "Impact of the Ebola
Epidemic on General and HIV Care in Macenta, Forest Guinea, 2014." *AIDS
(London, England)* 29, no. 14 (2015). https://www.ncbi.nlm.nih.gov/pmc
/articles/PMC4571280/.

Lewis, Maureen. "The Economics of Epidemics." *Georgetown Journal of International Affairs* 2, no. 2 (2001): 25–31. http://www.jstor.org/stable/43134024.

"Liberian Orphanages." *Guardian,* November 24, 2009. https://www.theguardian
.com/society/gallery/2009/nov/24/international-aid-and-development
-children.

Link, Bruce G., and Jo C. Phelan. "Conceptualizing Stigma." *Annual Review of
Sociology* 27, no. 1 (2001): 363–85. https://doi.org/10.1146/annurev.soc.27.1.363.

Long, Callie. "Fighting Fear and Stigma with Accurate Information." Health
Communication Capacity Collaborative. August 19, 2015. https://health
commcapacity.org/fighting-fear-and-stigma-with-accurate-information/.

MacDougall, Claire. "Fearing the Tide in West Point, a Slum Already Swamped
with Worry." New York Times, March 16, 2016. https://www.nytimes.com
/2016/03/16/world/africa/fearing-the-tide-in-west-point-a-slum-already
-swamped-with-worry.html.

Macrotrends. "Freetown, Sierra Leone Metro Area Population 1950–2021." July
2023. www.macrotrends.net/cities/22445/freetown /population.

Macrotrends. "Monrovia, Liberia Metro Area Population 1950–2021." July 2023.
https://www.macrotrends.net/cities/21779/monrovia/population.

Maddi, Salvatore. "Personal Hardiness as the Basis for Resilience." In *Hardiness:
Turning Stressful Circumstances into Resilient Growth,* ed. Salvatore Maddi.
Springer, Dordrecht, 2013, 7–17.

Markel, Howard. " 'Knocking out the Cholera': Cholera, Class, and Quarantines
in New York City, 1892." *Bulletin of the History of Medicine* 69, no. 3 (1995):
420–57. https://www.jstor.org/stable/44451706.

Masten, Ann, and Jelena Obradovic. "Disaster Preparation and Recovery: Lessons from Research on Resilience in Human Development." *Ecology and Society* 13, no. 1 (June 2008): 8–9. https://www.jstor.org/stable/26267914.

Matua, Gerald, and Rozanno Locsin. "Conquering Death From Ebola: Living the Experience of Surviving a Life-Threatening Illness." In *Coping With Disease,* 121–73. Nova Science, 2005.

Matua, Gerald Amandu, and Dirk Mostert Van der Wal. "Living Under the Constant Threat of Ebola: A Phenomenological Study of Survivors and Family Caregivers During an Ebola Outbreak." *Journal of Nursing Research* 23, no. 3 (2015): 217–24. https://doi.org/10.1097/jnr.0000000000000116.

Mayrhuber, Elisabeth Anne-Sophie, Thomas Niederkrotenthaler, and Ruth Kutalek. "'We Are Survivors and Not a Virus': Content Analysis of Media Reporting on Ebola Survivors in Liberia." *PLoS Neglected Tropical Diseases* 11, no. 8 (2017): e0005845. https://doi.org/10.1371/journal.pntd.0005845.

McFerson, Hazel. "Women and Post-Conflict Society in Sierra Leone." *Journal of International Women's Studies* 13, no. 1 (2012): 46–67. https://core.ac.uk/download/pdf/48828219.pdf.

Mehtar, Shaheen, Andre N.H. Bulabula, Haurace Nyandemoh, and Steve Jambawai. "Deliberate Exposure of Humans to Chlorine—The Aftermath of Ebola in West Africa." *Antimicrobial Resistance & Infection Control* 5, no. 1 (November 2016): 1–8. https://doi.org/10.1186/s13756-016-0144-1.

Missoni, Eduardo. "The political economy of epidemics." *Epidémies et sociétés, passé, présent et futur, Edizioni ETS* (2017): 171–90. https://asvis.it/public/asvis2/files/Approfondimenti/170623-Epidemics-and-Societies-The-political-economy-of-epidemics-proof.pdf.

Moncivais, Katy. "911 Victims Compensation." ConsumerSafety. Accessed 2023. https://www.consumersafety.org/resources/9-11-victim-compensation-fund/.

Mullan, Zoë. "The Cost of Ebola." *Lancet Global Health* 3, no. 8 (2015): e423. https://doi.org/10.1016/S2214-109X(15)00092-3.

National Institutes of Health. "Study Finds Ebola Survivors in Liberia Face Ongoing Health Issues." March 2019. https://www.nih.gov/news-events/news-releases/study-finds-ebola-survivors-liberia-face-ongoing-health-issues.

National Public Radio. "The Ebola Survivors Who Can't Go Home." October 2014. Transcript. https://www.npr.org/transcripts/357008487.

NBC News. "Why Has Nurse Amber Vinson Recovered from Ebola So Quickly?" NBC.com. 2014. https://www.nbcnews.com/storyline/ebola-virus-outbreak/why-has-nurse-amber-vinson-recovered-ebola-so-quickly-n232431.

Neria, Yuval, Priya Wickramaratne, Mark Olfson, et al. "Mental and Physical Health Consequences of the September 11, 2001 (9/11) Attacks in Primary

Care: A Longitudinal Study." *Journal of Traumatic Stress* 26, no. 1 (2013): 45–55. https://doi.org/10.1002/jts.21767.

Neufeld, Edward. "Hygiene Conditions in Ancient Israel (Iron Age)." *Journal of the History of Medicine and Allied Sciences* 25, no. 4 (1970): 414–37. https://doi.org/10.1093/jhmas/XXV.4.414.

Nigg, Joanne. *Disaster Recovery as a Social Process.* University of Delaware UDSPACE. Preliminary Paper no. 219. 1995. http://udspace.udel.edu/handle/19716/625.

Obeng-Odoom, Franklin, and Matthew Marke Beckhio Bockarie. "The Political Economy of the Ebola Virus Disease." *Social Change* 48, no. 1 (2018): 18–35. https://doi.org/10.1177/0049085717743832.

Ojha, Abin. "Is Pandemic a Class-Ridden? An Appraisal from New York City." *Journal of Ethnic and Cultural Studies* 7, no. 3 (2020): 129–41. https://doi.org/10.29333/ejecs/535.

Omonzejele, Peter. "Current Ethical and Other Problems in the Practice of African Traditional Medicine." *Medicine & Law* 22 (2003): 29–38. https://heinonline.org/HOL/LandingPage?handle=hein.journals/mlv22&div=7&id=&page=.

Onwujekwe, Obinna, Prince Agwu, Charles Orjiakor, et al. "Corruption in Anglophone West Africa Health Systems: A Systematic Review of Its Different Variants and the Factors That Sustain Them." *Health Policy and Planning* 34, no. 7 (2019): 529–43. https://doi.org/10.1093/heapol/czz070.

Onyango, Monica Adhiambo, Kirsten Resnick, Alexandra Davis, and Rupal Ramesh Shah. "Gender-Based Violence Among Adolescent Girls and Young Women: A Neglected Consequence of the West African Ebola Outbreak." In *Pregnant in the Time of Ebola*, 121–32. Springer, Cham, 2019.

Overholt, Luc, David Alain Wohl, William A. Fischer, et al. "Stigma and Ebola Survivorship in Liberia: Results from a Longitudinal Cohort Study." *PLoS ONE* 13, no. 11 (2018): e0206595. https://doi.org/10.1371/journal.pone.0206595.

Partners in Health. "Blindness." February 2017. https://medium.com/partnersinhealth/blindness-651fa693700a.

Peterman, Amber. "Widowhood and Asset Inheritance in Sub-Saharan Africa: Empirical Evidence from 15 Countries." *Development Policy Review* 30, no. 5 (2012): 543–71. https://doi.org/10.1111/j.1467-7679.2012.00588.x.

Peters, Stephanie True. *Smallpox in the New World.* Benchmark Books, 2005.

Porter, Roy. "The Patient's View." *Theory and Society* 14, no. 2 (1985): 175–98. https://doi.org/10.1007/BF00157532.

Rabelo, Ionara, Virginia Lee, Mosoka P. Fallah, et al. "Psychological Distress Among Ebola Survivors Discharged from an Ebola Treatment Unit in Monrovia, Liberia—A Qualitative Study." *Frontiers in Public Health* 4 (2016): 142. https://doi.org/10.3389/fpubh.2016.00142.

Reid, Megan. "Disasters and Social Inequalities." *Sociology Compass* 7, no. 11 (2013): 984. https://doi.org/10.1111/soc4.12080.

Reuters Staff. "DRC: Last Ebola Patient Discharged with End of Outbreak in Sight." Reuters. March 3, 2020. https://www.reuters.com/article/us-health-ebola-congo/last-congo-ebola-patient-discharged-with-end-of-outbreak-in-sight-idUSKBN20Q2B0.

Ribacke, Kim, Alex J. van Duinen, Helena Nordenstedt, et al. "The Impact of the West Africa Ebola Outbreak on Obstetric Health Care in Sierra Leone." *PLOS One*, 11, no. 2 (February 2016): e0150080. https://doi.org/10.1371/journal.pone.0150080.

Richards, Paul. *Ebola. How a People's Science Helped End an Epidemic*. Zed Books, 2016, 29–30.

Richards, Paul, Joseph Amara, Mariane C. Ferme, et al. "Social Pathways for Ebola Virus Disease in Rural Sierra Leone, and Some Implications for Containment." *PLoS Neglected Tropical Diseases* 9, no. 4 (April 2015): e0003567. https://doi.org/10.1371/journal.pntd.0003567.

Richardson, Eugene T., Mohamed Bailor Barrie, Cameron T. Nutt, et al. "The Ebola Suspect's Dilemma." *Lancet Global Health* 5, no. 3 (2017): e254–e256. https://doi.org/10.1016/S2214-109X(17)30041-4.

Riedel, Stefan. "Edward Jenner and the History of Smallpox and Vaccination." *Baylor University Medical Center Proceedings* 18, no. 1 (2005): 21–25. https://doi.org/10.1080/08998280.2005.11928028.

Root, Rebbeca L. "After Ebola Funds Fiasco, IFRC Is 'Confident' Corruption Won't Get COVID-19 Money." Devex. April 2020. https://www.devex.com/news/after-ebola-funds-fiasco-ifrc-is-confident-corruption-won-t-get-covid-19-money-96876.

Ryan, Sadie J., and Peter D. Walsh. "Consequences of Non-Intervention for Infectious Disease in African Great Apes." *PLOS One* 6, no. 12 (2011): e29030. https://doi.org/10.1371/journal.pone.0029030.

Santosa, Ailiana, Stig Wall, Edward Fottrell, Ulf Högberg, and Peter Byass. "The Development and Experience of Epidemiological Transition Theory over Four Decades: A Systematic Review." *Global Health Action* 7, no. 1 (2014): 23574. https://doi.org/10.3402/gha.v7.23574.

Schwerdtle, Patricia M., Veronique De Clerck, and Virginia Plummer. "Experiences of Ebola Survivors: Causes of Distress and Sources of Resilience." *Prehospital and Disaster Medicine* 32, No. 3 (2017): 234–39. https://doi.org/10.1017/S1049023X17000073.

Scott, Janet T., Foday R. Sesay, Thomas A. Massaquoi, Baimba R. Idriss, Foday Sahr, and Malcolm G. Semple. "Post-Ebola Syndrome, Sierra Leone." *Emerging Infectious Diseases* 22, no. 4 (2016): 641–46. https://doi.org/10.3201/eid2204.151302.

Secor, Andrew, Rose Macauley, Laurentiu Stan, et al. "Mental Health Among
 Ebola Survivors in Liberia, Sierra Leone and Guinea: Results from a Cross-
 Sectional Study." *BMJ Open* 10, no. 5 (2020): e035217. https://doi.org/10.1136
 /bmjopen-2019-035217.
Shantha, Jessica, Ian Crozier, and Steven Yeh. "An Update on Ocular Complications of Ebola Virus Disease." *Current Opinion in Ophthalmology* 28, no. 6
 (2017): 600–606. https://doi.org/10.1097/ICU.0000000000000426.
Shehu, Rezarta. "Social Police Regarding the Transformation of Family." *Journal
 of Educational and Social Research* 3, no. 3 (2013): 271–74. https://doi.org/10
 .5901/jesr.2013.v3n3p271.
"Sierra Leone: Grant-in-Aid Award, Students Cry Foul." *Standard Times*, March
 20, 2022. https://allafrica.com/stories/200203200429.html.
Sindzingre, Alice. "Theoretical Criticisms and Policy Optimism: Assessing the
 Debates on Foreign Aid." University of Vienna Department of Development
 Studies Working Paper 1. 2012. https://ie.univie.ac.at/fileadmin/user_upload
 /p_ie/INSTITUT/Publikationen/IE_Publications/ieWorkingPaper/IE-WP
 -1-2012_Sindzingre.pdf.
Snyder, Robert, Mariel Marlow, and Lee Riley. "Ebola in Urban Slums: The Ele-
 phant in the Room." *Lancet Global Health*, 2, no. 12 (December 2014): e685.
 https://doi.org/10.1016/S2214-109X(14)70339-0.
Social Security Administration. "Liberia." 2019. https://www.ssa.gov/policy/docs
 /progdesc/ssptw/2018-2019/africa/liberia.html.
S.O.S. Children's Villages. "General Information on Sierra Leone." Accessed May
 2022. https://www.sos-childrensvillages.org/where-we-help/africa/sierra
 -leone#:~:text=According%20to%20estimates%2C%20310%2C000%20
 children,been%20orphaned%20due%20to%20AIDS.
Stein, Zena A., Jack Ume Tocco, Joanne E. Mantell, and Raymond A. Smith. "To
 Hasten Ebola Containment, Mobilize Survivors." *International Journal of
 Epidemiology* 43, no. 6 (2014): 1679–80. https://doi.org/10.1093/ije/dyu233.
Steptoe, Paul J., Nicholas A.V. Beare, Alimamy D. Fornah, Fayiah Momorie,
 Patrick Komba, Matthew Vandy, et al. "Visual Disability in Ebola Survivors."
 Clinical Infectious Diseases 66, no.8 (April 2018): 1318–19. https://doi.org
 /10.1093/cid/cix979.
Stock, Robert. *Africa South of the Sahara: A Geographical Interpretation.* 2nd ed.
 Guildford Press, 2004, 241.
Summers, Aimee, Tolbert G. Nyenswah, Joel M. Montgomery, John Neatherlin,
 and Jordan W. Tappero. "Challenges in Responding to the Ebola Epidemic—
 Four Rural Counties, Liberia, August–November 2014." *Morbidity and Mor-
 tality Weekly Report* 63, no. 50 (December 2014): 1202–4. https://pubmed
 .ncbi.nlm.nih.gov/25522089/.
Sutmoller, Paul, Simon S. Barteling, Raul Casas Olascoaga, and Keith J. Sump-

tion. "Control and Eradication of Foot-and-Mouth Disease." *Virus Research* 91, no. 1 (2003): 101–44. https://doi.org/10.1016/S0168–1702(02)00262–9.

Takahashi, Saki, C. Jessica E. Metcalf, Matthew J. Ferrari, et al. "Reduced Vaccination and the Risk of Measles and Other Childhood Infections Post-Ebola." *Science* 347, no. 6227 (2015): 1240–42. https://doi.org/10.1126/science .aaa3438.

Taylor, Robert, Linda Chatters, Christina J. Cross, and Dawne Mouzon. "Fictive Kin Networks Among African Americans, Black Caribbeans, And Non-Latino Whites." *Journal of Family Issues* 43, no. 1 (2022): 20–46. https://doi .org/10.1177/0192513X21993188.

Tierney, Kathleen, and Anthony Oliver-Smith. "Social Dimensions of Disaster Recovery." *International Journal of Mass Emergencies & Disasters* 30, no. 2 (2012): 123–46. https://doi.org/10.1177/028072701203000210.

United Nations News Center. "West African Communities Receiving Ebola's Orphans with Open Arms, UN Agency Reports." UN News. February 6, 2015. https://news.un.org/en/story/2015/02/490402-west-african-communities -receiving-ebolas-orphans-open-arms-un-agency-reports.

Van Bortel, Tine, Anoma Basnayake, Fatou Wurie, et al. "Psychosocial Effects of an Ebola Outbreak at Individual, Community and International Levels." *Bulletin of the World Health Organization* 94, no. 3 (2016): 210. https://doi .org/10.2471/BLT.15.158543.

Van Griensven, Johan, Tansy Edwards, Xavier de Lamballerie, et al. "Evaluation of Convalescent Plasma for Ebola Virus Disease in Guinea." *New England Journal of Medicine* 374, no. 1 (2016): 33–42. https://doi.org/10.1056/NEJMoa 1511812.

Virk, Jasmine. "Victim or Advocate? Conceptualising Biocitizenship in Recipients of Medical Humanitarian Intervention During South Africa's HIV/AIDS Epidemic." *Postgraduate Journal of Medical Humanities* (2020): 80–110. https://humanities.exeter.ac.uk/media/universityofexeter/collegeofhuman ities/history/researchcentres/centreformedicalhistory/pdfsanddocs/Victim _or_Advocate_-_.

White, Howard, Tony Killick, and Steve Kayizzi-Mugerwa. *African Poverty at The Millennium: Causes, Complexities, and Challenges.* World Bank Publications, 2001.

Wilson, Himiede W., Maame Amo-Addae, Ernest Kenu, Olayinka Stephen Ilesanmi, Donne K. Ameme, and Samuel O. Sackey. "Post-Ebola Syndrome Among Ebola Virus Disease Survivors in Montserrado County, Liberia 2016." *BioMed Research International* (January 2018). https://doi.org/10.1155/2018 /1909410.

World Bank. "Physicians (per 1,000 People)." Accessed June 15, 2023. https://data .worldbank.org/indicator/SH.MED.PHYS.ZS.

World Health Organization. "End of the Most Recent Ebola Virus Disease
    Outbreak in Liberia." June 9, 2016. https://www.who.int/news/item/09
    -06–2016-end-of-the-most-recent-ebola-virus-disease-outbreak-in-liberia.
World Health Organization. "Improving Access to Mental Health Services in
    Sierra Leone." August 2016. https://www.afro.who.int/news/improving
    -access-mental-health-services-sierra-leone.
Yadav, Sankalp, and Gautam Rawal. "The Current Mental Health Status of Ebola
    Survivors in Western Africa." *Journal of Clinical and Diagnostic Research* 9,
    no. 10 (2015): LA01–LA02. https://doi.org/10.7860/JCDR/2015/15127.6559.
Zapotoczny, Walter. "The Political and Social Consequences of the Black Death,
    1348–1351." Accessed June 10, 2023. http://www.wzaponline.com/yahoo_site
    _admin/assets/docs/ BlackDeath.292130639.pdf.

Index